HOW NOT TO DIE

Surprising Lessons on Living Longer, Safer, and Healthier
from America's Favorite Medical Examiner

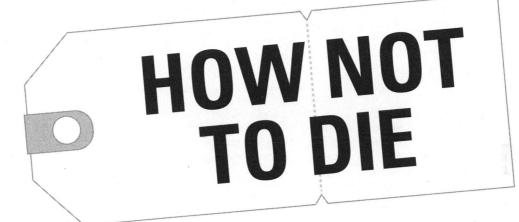

HOW NOT TO DIE

JAN GARAVAGLIA, M.D.

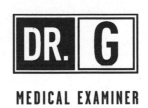

MEDICAL EXAMINER

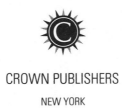

CROWN PUBLISHERS

NEW YORK

This book contains general information, including simple preventative measures
and lifestyle tips, on how to live a longer, healthier life.
It is not intended as a substitute for the advice and care of your physician,
and you should use proper discretion, in consultation with your physician,
in utilizing the information presented. The author and the publisher
expressly disclaim responsibility for any adverse effects that may result from
the use or application of the information contained in this book.

Copyright © 2008 by Atlas Media Corp. and Jan Garavaglia, M.D.

All rights reserved.
Published in the United States by Crown Publishers,
an imprint of the Crown Publishing Group,
a division of Random House, Inc., New York.
www.crownpublishing.com

CROWN and the Crown colophon are
registered trademarks of Random House, Inc.

The American Lung Association information in chapter 8 is reprinted with permission
© 2008 American Lung Association. For more information about the American Lung
Association or to support the work it does, call 1-800-LUNG-USA (1-800-586-4872)
or log on to www.lungusa.org.

Library of Congress Cataloging-in-Publication Data
Garavaglia, Jan.
How not to die : surprising lessons on living longer, safer, and healthier
from America's favorite medical examiner / Jan Garavaglia.
p. cm.
1. Garavaglia, Jan.   2. Medical examiners (Law)—United States—Biography.
3. Forensic pathology.   4. Self-care, Health.   I. Title.
RA1025.G33A3 2008
614'.1—dc22   2008027693

ISBN 978-0-307-40914-0

Printed in the United States of America

Design by Ruth Lee-Mui

2 4 6 8 9 7 5 3 1

First Edition

To my loving and steadfast husband, Mark Wallace,
and our three wonderful sons, Alex, Eric, and Luke

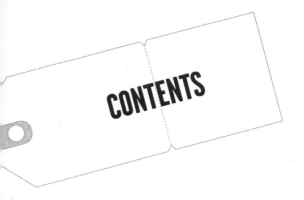

CONTENTS

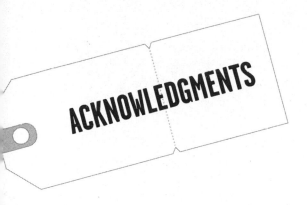

ACKNOWLEDGMENTS

To each and every decedent I have autopsied: I would like to thank you for the privilege of allowing me to learn from you. I'll never take that privilege for granted.

Mark Wallace: You are one of the most caring and intelligent physicians I have ever known and an even better husband and friend. Your collaboration on this book was invaluable and fun. Just like childbirth, I'm sure only the positive memories of the process will endure.

Maggie Greenwood-Robinson: I was lucky to have you as a partner on this project. You are a true professional. Your ability to translate ideas, concepts, and medical information into words is unparalleled, and your enthusiasm and optimism are infectious.

Bruce David Klein, the head of Atlas Media and producer of my show: You deserve a special thank-you. Your vision, inspiration, and drive were essential to this project. Your outstanding production staff at Atlas Media is wonderful to work with and does a terrific job in taking my stories about death and bringing them to life. I would especially like to thank Lorri Leighton, Cheryl Miller Houser, and my "Orlando crew" of Fahad Vania, Bobby Monahan, Adam Showen, and Andy Montejo for their outstanding performances and for making our work fun.

Craig Coffman, the original producer of the *Dr. G* series at Atlas Media: You also need a special thank-you because you were the reason I agreed to the pilot and series. Your sensitivity to the subject matter and, most important, the fact that you understood that everyone I autopsied had a story to tell, were crucial to the genesis of the series.

Discovery Health: Thank you for the privilege of my appearing on your network and being associated with such a quality organization. A special thanks to all the loyal fans of the *Dr. G* series who have supported the show for the past five years.

Heather Jackson, Heather Proulx, and the entire staff at Crown Publishers: I had heard wonderful things about you prior to writing this book, and you exceeded my expectations for creative input, insightful suggestions, and artful editing. Thank you all so much for working with me as part of your amazing team.

Everyone at the District Nine Medical Examiner's office: You deserve a big thank-you. Your support and tolerance of the show, as well as your compassion and professionalism, make the show and this book possible. Steve Hansen, my chief investigator, friend, and confidant, helps me keep things in perspective by causing me to laugh at the world, myself, and (mostly) him. Sheri Blanton is the world's greatest medical examiner's office administrator. Without you, none of this could have been possible. I greatly value your friendship, support, and confidence.

Eric Kowaleski: I know much of the time I spent on the book took you away from family fun, and I appreciate your indulgence. Alex Kowaleski: Thank you for being such a good sport about opening your life to the public. You're both wonderful sons.

My mother and family: Thank you for your love and support. And to my new family in Washington: Thank you for your acceptance and for loaning Mark to me.

HOW NOT TO DIE

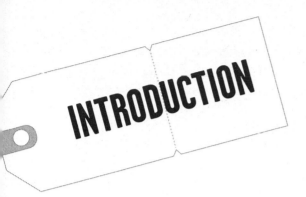

Confessions of a Real-Life Forensic Pathologist

Something was lodged in her windpipe. As I probed with my gloved fingers, I discovered that it was a piece of gum. Normally, this wouldn't be odd, except that I found it in a cadaver I was dissecting as a first-year medical student. Cadavers are preserved hulls of bodies, donated remains. Doctors-to-be become acquainted with them in anatomy classes. To us, they aren't people. We learn to depersonalize our cadavers, to think of them as structures and tissues, not as human beings. And in med school, they're used to teach us anatomy, not how to find the cause of death. Cadavers don't usually give up clues. That's not their job.

But when this one died, she was chewing gum. This made me curious. How did she get to this point? Where did she come from? How did she die? I started asking if anyone could get me some history on my cadaver. The body, it turned out, was of a nun who died suddenly of cardiac arrest while chewing gum.

And so began my fascination with how people die.

I might as well take a moment here to introduce myself. I'm a medical examiner, the only type of doctor whose patients are dead. "Dr. G" is the nickname I was given by my team of autopsy technicians in Bexar County, Texas, where I served as medical examiner for ten years. My Italian last name, Garavaglia, is hard to pronounce correctly, since the second "g" is silent, like it is in "lasagna." My technicians shortened it to "Dr. G," and it stuck.

Like that "g," my patients are silent. They can't tell me how they died, so I have to find out. Their bodies store secrets and have stories to tell. Sometimes there aren't many details, maybe not even firm answers. But usually there are clues about how people lived, what diseases and injuries they had, and how they died. Those clues get discovered through an autopsy, a thorough, methodical examination of a body. The results can help solve crimes, settle lawsuits, and give families needed information about their loved ones. Often it is tricky work, like solving a puzzle.

During an autopsy, I make notes and take photographs. I do an internal examination organ by organ. I slice them into neat pieces with a carving knife, looking for irregularities. I've been told, "I could use you when I butcher a deer." But when I cut, I'm looking for answers. During the autopsy, I may make microscopic slides and take fluid samples for the toxicology laboratory. This is the methodology for finding out how someone died.

Preventing Premature Death

I obviously have no problems with autopsies, although I hope to wait a long time before one is conducted on me. I learn something from every one of them, and what I have discovered is that many deaths don't need to happen. Yes, everyone eventually dies. You can't prevent that, but you can avoid life's inevitable toe tag from arriving *prematurely.* And you can do it with the simplest lifesaving acts, whether it's strapping on a seat belt correctly, making subtle changes to your diet, or following your doctor's orders. That's not all, either. There are other actions you might not be aware of that can save your life. For example, did you know that open or partially open car windows increase the risk of more severe injuries in an accident? There are many lessons that can be learned from the dead—lessons that can help us, the living, take better care of ourselves. I wrote this book to show you how to avoid an early trip to the morgue.

I see ways to prevent premature death, just like other doctors see ways to prevent illness, and I'll share them with you on every page of this book. Through what I've seen and experienced, I will give you a new understanding of your health and the consequences of the everyday decisions you make, so you can take better care of yourself and everyone around you. Sure, your body may have a few dings and dents, but this body of yours has many more miles to go, too. I've organized the book around topics to bring you better health, such as losing weight, overcoming addiction, avoiding accidents, and surviving a hospital stay. Clearly, some accidents are unavoidable and some sudden natural deaths are inevitable, but the simple measures outlined here will give you an edge.

The dead and their autopsies have been great teachers for me, but not until I started taping my television show, *Dr. G: Medical Examiner,* did I realize that others could also be moved to action by my stories from the morgue. Many times, a televised case will generate letters and comments from viewers who finally make the concrete connection between their behaviors and their health. They see the evidence of the harmful things we do to our bodies: lungs mottled with black streaks due to smoking, organs dangerously enlarged by obesity, arteries choked off by plaque, and once brown, healthy livers turned yellow and fatty from alcohol abuse. The body tells the tale of how someone lived, how they died, and how that death might have been prevented.

A lot of people argue that when death comes, "it's your time to die." I don't believe the difference between life and death always turns on timing. Sure, some people just have bad luck and develop an illness or suffer an accident that is totally unavoidable, but a lot of us make our own bad luck. Life is a series of choices. And these choices, plus genetics and luck, determine our fate. You can control what you eat, you can control how fast you drive, you can control whether or not you abuse drugs—you control the choices you make. Making the right choices can offer a chance at a much longer and healthier life.

I remember doing an autopsy on an old man found facedown in the dirt next to his back porch with contused and bloody hands. (You'll read more about this case in chapter 9.) At first, it looked like this man was possibly the victim of foul play. But the autopsy and scene investigation revealed a man suffering from dementia who became confused after retrieving his mail. He tore his screen door, cut his hands, slipped, and fell.

What could anyone learn about healthy choices from the death of this man who had the misfortune of having Alzheimer's, as of today an unpreventable disease? When performing this seemingly routine autopsy, I took the opportunity to show my producer how our Western diet, with its lack of fiber, had ravaged this man's colon by causing diverticulitis—small pouches in the wall of the colon had become inflamed. The appearance of that colon had a profound effect on my producer when I explained the reason for these changes was lack of fiber and exercise, causing the stool to move slowly through the bowel and creating increased pressure in the bowel lumen. Suddenly the light went on. My producer understood why his own doctor had been telling him to increase his fiber intake and exercise. Prior to seeing that bowel, it was empty advice, but combined with that visual, it motivated him to change.

Through my work with the dead, I've often seen untreated illnesses that get horribly out of control and cause premature and unexpected death. I still get comments about a case that aired on the *Dr. G* show in which an overweight middle-aged man, who lived alone and never bothered with a checkup, one day lumbered up the stairs to his second-floor apartment, groceries in hand, and when he went in, he sat down and died. The autopsy showed long-standing changes in his heart and kidneys and a large new bleed inside his brain, all caused by high blood pressure, an easily treated disease of which he was unaware. People tell me that that story motivated them to take their antihypertensive pills each day and get their blood pressure tested regularly, because they finally understood that high blood pressure is a silent killer.

Just as I tell students when I lecture on drugs and alcohol, I may not be an expert on *why* you decide to take drugs, or *how* to treat drug addiction, but I'm an expert on how drugs and alcohol cause you to end up in my morgue. If you choose to use drugs and abuse alcohol, you need to be aware of how they can and do kill. Similarly, not watching your weight, not taking time to exercise, and eating junk food are choices you consciously make, and you should know the ultimate consequences of these decisions and how they might result in a quicker-than-expected trip to see me.

My Life in Forensics

The world of death and grieving families is probably not the life my parents would have imagined for me, but I love it. I love putting the pieces together, being able to use creative thought, and solving the mystery of death. When people ask me how I ended up in this line of work, I tell them about Dr. George Gantner, a prominent forensic pathologist and one of the founders of the specialty. I took a course from him in medical school and was riveted by what he did. His lectures, punctuated by all sorts of autopsy photos, were intriguing. When I chatted with him, I became even more fascinated with the work.

Dr. Gantner shaped my decision to become a forensic pathologist, but it was my high school chemistry teacher who inspired me to become a doctor. He told me I was capable of success in medicine, a field I found fascinating but had not previously considered. So I shelved my original plans to teach home economics. In thinking about a future career, I decided the two most-needed professions in society were farming and medicine. If the world starts falling apart, we need farmers to feed us and doctors to fix us. Since every plant I touched died, I said, Okay, I'll be a doctor.

As a young med student, I thought medicine was a noble profession, and I still do. But I got disillusioned as an intern and realized it might not suit my personality. I loved the workings of the human body, and I loved coming up with diagnoses. But dealing with patients' complaints day in and day out—so many complaints that were related to how they were living their lives—wore on me. At the time, I worked in a clinic where I treated people mostly for lifestyle-related conditions due to smoking, not exercising, being overweight, or alcohol consumption. Even though I'd prescribe medication and other treatments to help them, they'd return to the clinic month after month with the same complaints, and many weren't even taking their medicine. It frustrated me. I decided I couldn't keep that up for a lifetime.

As I investigated the field of forensic pathology, I worried that I wouldn't be contributing to society and that I'd be wasting my medical education. I came to realize, though, that you can do good in the world through forensics. Maybe you couldn't do anything for the individual you were examining, but you could help family members and society as a whole. Some families can't complete the grieving process with unanswered questions. Often I have family members say, "It can't be a suicide," for example. No one wants to believe a loved one would take his or her own life. Once I was called to autopsy an apparent suicide victim whose parents were very religious and believed that suicide was a sin. After doing the autopsy, I discovered that the deceased had died a natural death, from a brain aneurysm. The family was deeply grateful for that answer. On another occasion, a young man was brought to my morgue, and everyone thought he had died of a drug overdose. But his mother insisted that he did not do drugs. We repeated the toxicology tests and found that his mother was right. There was no evidence of drug use. Knowing how a family member died brings closure and comfort even if the answer is not what the loved ones want to hear. Though the information does not bring back a loved one, it does help the grieving process, and this is the healing I can give.

Forensic Pathology 101

My line of work is known as forensic pathology. It's the field of medicine concerned with how people die and ultimately determining the cause and manner of death. "Cause of death" refers to the action or condition that results in death and can include such things as suffocation, drowning, heart attack or stroke, gunshot wound, or a blow to the head or other body part. In contrast, "manner of death" refers to whether the death is the result of natural or unknown causes, homicide, suicide, or an accident.

It's hard for me to generalize about what I look for when deciphering a death, since every case is a mystery, but I do look at each one as though foul play could have happened and try to rule it out. A gunshot wound, for example, can be a suicide, a homicide, or an accident. With a gunshot, I'd ask, "Is it a weird angle? Is it a contact wound?" What the person left behind can tell me what happened; I'll see if the autopsy findings can confirm or deny what's been alleged. For example, a wife may say her husband had been despondent for weeks and finally got a gun and killed himself. I'd look at the wound to determine if it's a contact wound, which most suicides are, or whether it is the result of a gun fired from ten feet away. I've handled cases where everybody bought the story from the "grieving widow" until it was proven there was no way the husband could have pulled the trigger himself.

I'm Not a Coroner

There are two types of death investigation systems in the United States: coroner systems and medical examiner systems. At present, twelve states have coroner systems, nineteen have state medical examiner systems, three states have county or regional M.E. offices with no coroner offices, and sixteen have a mixture of medical examiner and coroner systems. It's a real patchwork.

I've often been asked if I'm a coroner. I explain that, no, I'm not a coroner, I'm also not a mortician, and I don't drive a hearse. Coroners are elected officials, and they usually aren't forensic pathologists. A coroner's training can range from absolutely none to full training in forensic pathology. A coroner could be a funeral home director, a tow-truck driver, or a CEO. In some states, anyone who runs for coroner and is elected gets the job. I've dealt with sheriffs who were coroners. I believe this is a conflict of interest. What would happen if someone died while in the sheriff's custody? The sheriff certainly wouldn't want suspicion cast on his department. What would be the public perception if he ruled the death as natural, regardless of whether his ruling was correct?

In making rulings, coroners don't have to consult physicians for advice, but they have to hire physicians to do autopsies. Even then, someone who is unfamiliar with signs of violence, for example, might confuse gunshot entrance and exit wounds or be unable to tell whether brain trauma was caused by a blow or a fall.

A coroner need not rule in agreement with autopsy findings. I have worked with coroners who are completely unqualified to rule on cause and manner of death. In some egregious cases, coroners have rejected forensic pathologists' findings of homicide and instead labeled deaths as "accidental," perhaps letting a few people get away with murder.

In fighting crime or deciphering a death, the most important clues are often furnished by the autopsy—which is why the best death investigation systems have an independent, well-trained forensic pathologist to investigate and certify deaths. Citizens deserve an honest voice, someone with no dog in the fight and who isn't subject to pressure, political or otherwise. As a medical examiner, I'm not beholden to the state attorney, law enforcement, or the hospital, because sometimes my decisions may have to go against any of them.

The coroner system, the older of the two death investigation systems, started with good intentions. The term "coroner" dates all the way back to the twelfth century A.D., to England. Back then, the sheriffs, who were the dominant law officers representing the Crown, were charged with collecting legal fines and taxes from the people and delivering them to the king. Instead, they extorted, embezzled, and basically did anything they could to keep the money for themselves. Once the king realized this, he set up a checks-and-balances system by appointing a coroner, or a keeper of the pleas of the Crown, to record everything that happened in the towns and cities throughout the country.

In those days, there were huge fines associated with death. (For example, say your ox cart rolled over my son. The sheriffs would confiscate your ox and cart and some of your possessions as payback, and a cut of that would go to the king.) So one of the coroner's most important functions became the recording of death and everything relating to it—the circumstances; the cause; the what, where, when, and why. This is pretty similar to my job today.

Massachusetts was the first state to institute a medical examiner system, in 1877, when lay coroners were replaced by physicians who were empowered to determine cause and manner of death. Until 1940, the Massachusetts medical examiner did not have the right to order autopsies. But the law was eventually changed, allowing autopsies at the discretion of the medical examiner.

The first modern medical examiner system was established in New York City in 1918, when the city adopted a law that abolished the coroner system. A physician with experience in pathology was appointed chief medical examiner and could perform autopsies without family consent. Medical examiner systems don't always run smoothly. New York City's system was crippled in the 1980s by the enactment of a law that allowed families to stop autopsies in cases in which the manner of death didn't appear to be homicide. That's a problem, since you can't always recognize a homicide until you do an autopsy. Thankfully, that law has been modified.

Inside My Morgue

Often I'm asked how I deal with the loss of human life and with loved ones. I grew up as the only daughter of an Italian butcher from St. Louis, Missouri. Death has never really bothered me. I see it as a natural part of life. I was brought up Catholic, with a set of clear moral values. Although I was taught that there's a heaven and a hell, I didn't put much thought into what happens to us after we die. But I don't believe that we go through this world just to end up on a slab. You can look at the faces of the dead and you know something is missing. It's the soul, and it has departed from the body.

I've been a medical examiner for most of my adult life—one of about five hundred in the United States. Every year, my jurisdiction—District Nine of Orange County, Florida—performs more than eleven hundred painstaking autopsies, looking for the often-hidden signs of wounds, disease, or trauma.

Some people believe that forensic pathologists deal only with homicide victims or that the majority of our cases involve crime. The truth is that in my office, as in most medical examiners' offices in the United States, only around 10 percent of the cases are homicides. About 40 percent of the deaths that come through my office are from premature natural disease; 40 percent are accidents; and 10 percent are suicides. Based on those statistics, it's striking to me how many of the deaths I deal with are premature and could have been avoided with better lifestyle choices, preventive care, or commonsense caution.

The tools we use in the morgue are not the stuff of high-tech medicine like you'd see in a hospital, since our job isn't to bring people back to life. It's to solve the mystery of what happened to them. We use a lot of familiar household-type objects: carving knives, knife sharpeners, hedge clippers, and sponges with scouring pads on one side, in addition to our normal tools of the trade like scalpels and bone saws. I've even used superglue (about $2.69 at the drugstore) to bring the edges of a wound back together so I could see its characteristics more clearly. We have a large walk-in refrigerator in the morgue, too, like the kind you see in restaurants. We use it to slow down decomposition. The back shelves of our cooler are for our "long-term residents," the unidentified bodies we hold while their identities are being investigated.

Present during an autopsy are the medical examiners, who are all doctors, and our technicians, who assist us. From time to time, others drop by, like detectives working a case. I don't usually allow people to observe an autopsy unless there is good reason. The people I work on didn't ask to be there and probably wouldn't appreciate an audience.

Once, my son Alex, four years old at the time, accidentally wandered into the autopsy suite while I was performing an autopsy. He saw the skull and brain resting on the sink. I was horrified but quickly composed myself and vowed not to make a big deal of it. I explained what I was doing in matter-of-fact language, so he could see that it was my job. He watched for a moment, then asked, "Can I leave?"

For the next few days, I watched for repercussions like nightmares, but Alex seemed fine. Then I heard what he was saying at nursery school when kids asked him what his mom did for a living. He'd tell them, "She cuts off people's heads."

After doing an autopsy, I retreat to my desk, which is badly in need of a bulldozer, and dictate a report. It's transcribed by medical transcriptionists and will be read by many people. This is detail work essential to my job, but scarcely the stuff of drama. I sign a death certificate and make sure the body gets to the right place. I share my findings with the family members, who are understandably eager to know how their loved one passed.

What I do is interesting to people, and that's why TV shows depicting this work are so popular. Forensic stories are always fascinating, whether they're real or created in drama. For me, it's always the real stories that are most interesting. Fiction rarely holds my interest because I feel that the stories or the cases I work on every day are more interesting. Sometimes you can't make up the things that happen because nobody would believe them.

My show, *Dr. G: Medical Examiner,* deals with the real stories, but we use dramatizations to re-create them. When they show a dead body, it's an actor, out of respect to the families. Even if the families give permission, it's very hard to see a dead loved one on the screen. Being sensitive to the families is part of my job.

As a forensic pathologist, I see a lot of things that most people don't—deaths that shouldn't have happened, deaths that are senseless tragedies, and more. It isn't always the traumatic or the dramatic that kills us, but the small lapses in attention and judgment made in an instant or imperceptibly over time that can do us in. I've come to appreciate that how we choose to live plays a vital role in our health and well-being. Surprisingly, being surrounded by death has taught me how to live a healthier, happier life, and I've changed my own behaviors as a result of what I see every day. I don't have all the answers and don't treat the living, but I have great insights into how not to die.

If there's one thing that working in a room of the prematurely dead has taught me, it is that life is precious, and you never know when it's going to be taken away. I'll never take for granted that I'm alive and healthy, and I plan on staying that way as long as I can. And I want to help you do the same.

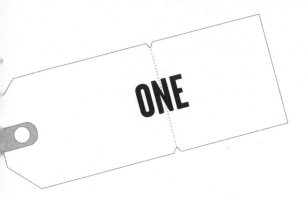

ONE

Doctor Dread

Taking It on the Jaw

I followed the infection underneath his breastbone like a trail of bread crumbs all the way up to his jaw. The trail teemed with pus, the army of white blood cells that had marched through the walls of blood vessels to fight invading microorganisms. I had never seen anything like it before. Bacteria had waged a protracted war with his body's immune system—and won. I wondered how fifty-year-old Victor Baca could have developed such a virulent infection.

Ten days earlier, Victor had been in perfect health. Then he started complaining of back and shoulder pain and a sore throat. The symptoms kept him in bed and unable to go to work. Even so, he didn't seek medical attention. But as the pain worsened, Victor realized something was terribly wrong, and he called 911. The dispatcher alerted an ambulance. Paramedics arrived, found him critically ill, and went to work immediately. Despite their aggressive intervention, including cardiopulmonary resuscitation (CPR), Victor slipped away, causes unknown.

As I often do in cases involving unusual infections, after the autopsy I consulted Dr. Mark Wallace, an infectious disease specialist and an internal medicine physician, who also happens to be my husband. An infectious disease specialist tracks down bacteria and viruses, decodes their defenses and their weaknesses, and figures out what will kill them. Mark believed—and I concurred—that all the evidence proved that a bacterial infection had originated in Victor's mouth, shockingly, from the most ordinary of health problems: a common dental infection.

This infection probably migrated from a decayed tooth into the surrounding bone and tissue in his jaw and caused an abscess, a cavity containing pus surrounded by inflamed tissue. Many of us have probably had an abscess at one time or another. They can show up externally (in the gums or in a hair follicle) or internally (in an organ), and some types are more severe than others.

Once a pocket of pus breaks through the thin bone surrounding the tooth sockets, bacteria can spread through the tissue planes of the neck and into the chest. By the time Victor sought medical attention, bacteria had likely reached his bloodstream and caused multisystem organ failure. This infection was the source of all his pain—and the cause of his death.

Before penicillin was discovered in 1928, bacterial infections like Victor's were the leading cause of death in the United States. Today, due to widespread use of antibiotics, head and neck infections rarely kill, unless you have no access to, or reject, basic medical or dental care. For some unknown reason, Victor decided not to see a doctor, even as the unchecked infection spread to his chest and the pain became excruciating. What began as a run-of-the-mill oral infection became a fight for survival. Eventually, Victor's organs ceased functioning, and he died. The tragedy was compounded by the fact that Victor's death could easily have been prevented. A routine course of antibiotics provided in a timely manner would have stopped the infection in its tracks.

Checked Out

As with the case of Victor Baca, I've seen firsthand the terrible complications that can arise when people don't go to the doctor, ignore a physician's advice, or decide to take medical matters into their own hands. Another example from my case files is that of Kim Atani, age forty-eight. She was a woman who could have lived a long, normal life had she received proper medical care. Kim, who was blind, and her husband, Simon, were living in their Orlando home when Simon found her collapsed on the bedroom floor. He called 911, and Kim was rushed to the hospital, where she later died. Her body was sent to my morgue to be autopsied.

Some of the most important information any physician—forensic pathologists included—can have is a medical history. But Kim arrived at the morgue without any medical records. I had to rely solely on observation to figure out why she died.

Clearly, something terrible had been happening. Her teeth were fractured at the gum line. She was also covered with bedsores, oozing craterlike wounds that can become seriously infected. Medically known as "decubitus ulcers," bedsores develop quickly as tissue dies when blood flow is impaired by the continuous pressure of body weight on the soft tissues sandwiched between bone and a firm surface. There was also gangrene, or dead tissue, which appeared as large, black, shriveled areas across her left foot. Gangrene is caused by progressive loss of blood to an area, and there are two types: wet and dry. Both are caused by poor blood flow, but in wet gangrene, the tissue is also infected with bacteria. Kim had wet gangrene. Gangrene is often associated with advanced cases of diabetes.

I dissected Kim's wet gangrene and discovered that the infection had burrowed down to her bone. If discovered in time, a limb so acutely diseased would have been amputated to prevent the spread of a life-threatening infection.

With my scalpel, I made the standard Y incision, a deep cut from shoulder to shoulder across the chest, followed by a straight line down to the pubic bone. I then opened the torso like you'd open a jacket or sport coat. Ribs were cut so I could gain access to the organs, which are removed, weighed, and dissected during the autopsy.

After opening her up, I could see that her body harbored several other possible killers. Her kidneys and liver were damaged, and her coronary arteries were more than 95 percent blocked. These findings were pieces of the puzzle that, along with her blindness, periodontal disease, and gangrene, began to fit a pattern. It appeared to me that Kim Atani had been suffering from long-standing untreated diabetes.

Diabetes is a metabolic disorder. Its hallmark is a failure to metabolize glucose, or blood sugar, carried by the bloodstream to fuel every part of the body. The failure is caused by problems with the hormone insulin. Either the body doesn't make any (or enough) insulin, or cells don't respond to insulin properly. In either situation, glucose is unable to enter cells. It starts amassing in the bloodstream, where it can reach concentrations over ten times the normal level. Over time, elevated glucose causes widespread organ damage, like that which I observed in Kim Atani.

To confirm that Kim had diabetes, I would need to know her blood sugar levels. Testing for blood sugar is easy to do when you're living—blood is drawn and checked for its glucose concentration—but it's more complicated when you're dead. After you die, your blood sugar begins to drop continuously toward zero. I can't even test for glucose levels in the blood because the blood breaks down right after death and interferes with testing. But I can test for glucose by using eye fluid drawn into a syringe—a procedure that can make you shudder if you've never seen it before. Each adult human eye contains about one-fifth of a teaspoon of jellylike fluid called vitreous humor. This fluid is very reliable for testing because it is isolated and protected, and therefore less subject to contamination or cell breakdown.

I collected eye fluid from Kim's eyes and sent it to our toxicology lab. Glucose levels in the eye decrease after death, too, so a finding of elevated glucose would strongly indicate diabetes. Sure enough, when the toxicology report came back, it revealed that Kim's eye-fluid glucose was 378—massively elevated for a postmortem level.

Once I put all the facts of the case together and reviewed her tissues under a microscope, it was clear to me that over time, elevated glucose had caused widespread organ disease. It not only left Kim blind but it also caused a loss of sensation in her extremities and impaired her blood flow. Gangrene set in and allowed a deadly infection to take hold. The infection invaded her bloodstream, causing sepsis—an often fatal condition.

Sepsis takes its name from the Greek word meaning "to putrefy." Known for generations as "blood poisoning," it generally means bacteria have breached the natural barriers of the skin and organs to enter the bloodstream. Once there, they produce an overwhelming infection, the biological equivalent of tossing a grenade into your body. Blood pressure drops, vessels leak, and the lungs and kidneys fail. The result can be septic shock so severe that no amount of intravenous fluid or medication can reverse the condition. This is what happened to Kim Atani.

Normally, a case like this would be closed, but I had to get to the bottom of why she had not sought medical care. Was it a case of negligence on the part of her husband, Simon? Could his inaction have contributed to her untimely death? If it was found that he had acted negligently, charges could be brought against him.

I called Simon and told him that his wife had had diabetes. He was in denial about it, but more from ignorance about the disease than anything else. I pointedly asked why she didn't seek medical care and why he didn't seek medical care for her. He told me that his wife had had some bad experiences with doctors, that she refused to see one, and that she hated the medical establishment. There was nothing he could do to get Kim to see a doctor, and so he vowed that he would do what he could to take care of her. In the end, and after confirming her fear of the medical system, I believed him. He was sincere and really cared about his wife.

Many people make choices that ultimately lead to their demise, and at autopsy, my findings reflect this. As a medical examiner, I'm one of the few people given permission to look behind the curtain of someone's life, and what I observe is often senseless and tragic. I don't judge how people live, but I will say this: Not going to the doctor when you have a major health issue is your decision, but missing needed care might mean I'll be the doctor you'll eventually visit.

Kim Atani and Victor Baca suffered not only from deadly but treatable illnesses; they also may have suffered from latrophobia or odontophobia. These are medical terms that describe a fear of doctors or dentists, respectively, in which people put off getting medical attention, making excuse after excuse, until sometimes it's too late.

Why do we fear doctors? I think one of the big reasons is that we're filled with dread that some serious problem might be found and we're afraid of hearing bad news. It's scary to be a patient. It's even scary for *me* to be a patient! Though we like to think we'll live forever, we're all here temporarily. Seeing a doctor brings us face-to-face with our own mortality.

There are other reasons we avoid seeing a doctor. Maybe you don't think your symptoms are important. Maybe you're concerned about wasting a doctor's time. Or maybe you don't want to spend the money because you're uninsured. I can't tell you how many people I've autopsied because they didn't want to incur a medical bill.

Or maybe you're a man. Men in this country are much less likely to see a doctor than women are. Their reluctance may be one reason why the life expectancy of men is eight years shorter than that of women. Men repress pain, ignore symptoms, and deny sickness, in part to demonstrate their manhood. Society conditions men to "tough out" illness. They don't want to feel like wimps or go to the doctor for nothing. If a man does see a doctor, it's often because a woman in his life has made him go.

How Not to Die from Latrophobia or Odontophobia

No one likes to get sick. It means that you can't do the things you enjoy or the things you live for. When you're sick, you don't feel like doing much of anything, except lying in bed. You might get better on your own, but then again, you might not. If you stay sick long enough, sooner or later you'll have to go to the doctor, whether you want to or not.

Wanted: A Great Doctor

If you're afraid of doctors, one of the best ways to get over your fear is to be under the care of one you like and trust. To find that kind of doctor takes a bit of sleuthing. Here's what I do: I look for a doctor who is geographically convenient, and I won't go to any doctor who is not board certified in his or her specialty or subspecialty. Board certification means that a doctor has had extra training after medical school and internship in an approved training program to become an expert in a field of medicine such as family practice, internal medicine, or gynecology, then has passed a rigorous qualifying examination ("the boards").

Personality is important to me, too, so I ask around to get a feel for what a doctor is like. Nurses are a great resource, since they're the ones who work with doctors day to day and see how they treat patients. I also ask friends, family, coworkers, and colleagues. Another good source is the website of the American Medical Association (www.ama-assn.org) with its DoctorFinder link. It gives you basic professional information on virtually every licensed physician in the United States. Of course, if you belong to a managed health-care plan, your choices are limited to doctors who are a part of that plan.

I also want a doctor who treats me with respect and doesn't sugarcoat things. What you need most is good communication. You end up telling a doctor a lot of intimate details about your life. If you feel uncomfortable doing so, that's your signal to find another one.

Here are ten questions to ask when choosing a new doctor:

1. Are you board certified in your specialty?
2. What type of health insurance do you take? (If applicable, find out if the doctor accepts Medicare.)
3. How frequently do you see patients who have the same health problems as I have?
4. Do you refer patients to other doctors for special problems as needed?
5. Will I need to go to another location for blood tests or are lab tests done in your office?
6. If yours is a group practice, who are the other doctors and what are their specialties?

7. Who sees patients for you if you are out of town or not available?

8. Which hospitals do you use? Will you take care of me in the hospital if I'm admitted? If not, who will? (Make sure you're comfortable being treated at one of these institutions, should the need arise.)

9. How far in advance do I need to make an appointment to see you?

10. If I've got a problem (say a drug reaction or a treatment side effect) can I speak to you or your covering physician within a reasonable time frame?

The M.D. or the M.E.?: When to See Your Doctor

It's not a good idea to rush off to the doctor for every little ache and pain, but many symptoms are signs that the situation could be serious. If you try to outlast your medical problems, you may be making more trips to a doctor in the long run or, worse yet, a trip to the morgue. Here's what happened when one of my patients passed his symptoms off as little more than the flu.

Murder or Malady?

Michael Peterson's body was about to be embalmed. Embalming is the centuries-old process by which a person is made to look alive after he's dead. Michael's blood would be drained and replaced by about four gallons of preservatives, his mouth would be wired shut, and since the eyes sink back into their sockets after death, cotton would be stuffed between his eyes and eyelids. Unlike Michael, you don't have to be embalmed after you die, unless there will be an open-casket ceremony. If you do your spadework, you'll find there are other options regarding your disposal. You can go the cremation route, in which your body is cooked at a temperature of around 2,500 degrees. On average, it takes an hour and a half for you to burn. Your ashes are returned to your loved ones in an urn, which can be displayed on the mantle or sprinkled over your garden. Whether you're embalmed and entombed or your ashes are fired from a cannon, the price tag for your funeral may run from $5,000 to $10,000. Disposing of their dead is, for many families, one of the most expensive purchases they will ever make, right behind buying a car or funding a college education.

Just as the morticians were ready to carry out Michael's funeral wishes, the phone rang. It was my office calling, ordering the funeral home to halt any and all procedures on the body. Surfacing like swamp bubbles were allegations that Michael had been murdered. Had Michael been embalmed, potential evidence would have been destroyed, and the autopsy would be more difficult.

Fifty-year-old Michael Peterson had been in the hospital, fighting to stay alive despite failing kidneys. Before illness struck, things had been looking up for this retired truck driver. He had just asked his ex-wife Katharine to marry him again, hoping to pick up where they'd left off fourteen years earlier. But their wedding was not to be. On the seventh day in the intensive care unit (ICU), with Katharine at his side, Michael lost his battle. The hospital recorded his death as natural, due to kidney disease.

But Michael's hospital roommate had a different opinion, and the next morning what he told the nurse changed everything. The roommate alleged that Katharine had murdered Michael. I couldn't ignore the allegations, so I decided to bring Michael's body in.

As his body was being transported to my morgue, I reviewed the details of the accusations. According to my investigator's report, the roommate heard some kind of gasping, as if Michael was struggling to breathe. Gradually the breathing became more ragged. The disturbing sound stopped suddenly. The roommate believed Katharine had smothered Michael with a pillow. He then claimed he saw Katharine rush past his bed and into the hallway. "She told the nurse, 'He's gone, he's gone,' and then ran out of the hospital."

According to the U.S. Department of Justice, almost 15 percent of all murders are committed by a member of the victim's family, a fact we know all too well in the morgue. The allegations sounded like they could have been credible, so I took them seriously. Michael's daughter told us that after the couple divorced, Katharine had never really left the picture. Their relationship was argumentative and stormy, further lending credence to the roommate's accusation. I began to wonder: Did Michael Peterson die of natural causes as the hospital believed, or did his ex-wife give Mother Nature a little push? Unlike the majority of autopsies I do, I would not cut open Michael Peterson's body to examine his internal organs. The hospital records contained enough information to show that Michael had died of acute kidney failure.

I would concentrate on the outside of the body in a search for signs of foul play.

The first thing I spotted was a huge bruise on the back of Michael's left shoulder. The mysterious injury was clearly not from the alleged murder, but I wanted to get to the bottom of it before continuing the exam. I returned to my investigator's report and discovered that there was more to Michael's story. He had been feeling ill, with some flu-like symptoms. On top of that, he had suffered an accidental fall four days before he was admitted to the hospital. The fall happened in the apartment he shared with his ex-wife.

Getting up from the couch, he felt faint and fell onto a coffee table, smashing his left shoulder. In terrible pain, he dragged himself over to the couch to lie down, and he remained there for four days, unable to get up and suffering from what he believed was simply the flu. Day in and day out, Michael's only sustenance were the ice cubes Katharine fed him, and that was the extent of the care he received. Eventually, he began drifting in and out of consciousness. Michael's back also had bedsores that had penetrated to the tissue underneath his skin.

Lying motionless on the couch for four days not only instigated Michael's bedsores but also triggered a potentially fatal condition called rhabdomyolysis, a fancy name for muscle breakdown. When you lie stationary for an extended period of time, your skeletal muscles can begin to physically deteriorate, especially muscles weakened by injury or the flu. As these muscles break down, the muscle cells release a protein called myoglobin that spills into the kidneys. Myoglobin wends its way through the meshwork of the kidney capillaries, accumulates in the tubules, and blocks the flow of fluid through the organs. The damaged kidneys can't filter toxic substances out of the body or regulate body chemistry. In Michael's case, these changes ultimately resulted in multiple organ failure.

Rhabdomyolysis, while occasionally fatal, is treatable in its early stages. Had Michael gotten medical care sooner, his condition could have been reversed.

I returned to the main reason for my examination—the hunt for physical evidence of suffocation that would prove Michael Peterson was murdered. I examined Michael's head and neck, looking for any kind of trauma. But I could find no such evidence. I knew that pillows are often used in suffocations because their soft surface leaves no marks on the body. At least that's what killers think. But suffocation can leave clues, literally right under the victim's nose. These clues can be pillow fibers or injuries in and around the mouth. But I could find nothing of the sort on Michael. There was no evidence that Michael was suffocated. Michael's hospital roommate, who I learned was sedated at the time, was wrong. Katharine did not murder her ex-husband. Most likely what the roommate heard behind the separation curtain were simply the last, labored gasps of a dying man.

My examination was finished, but one question remained unanswered. Why had Michael spent four days on his couch without getting medical attention, especially since his ex-wife was with him the whole time? Before long, my investigators uncovered the last remaining piece of the puzzle: an emergency response report filed just one day after Michael's fall. It revealed that Katharine, rather than acting neglectfully, had indeed called 911. Paramedics arrived and attempted to take Michael to the ER but he refused, insisting that he merely had a flu bug. Legally, emergency medical teams aren't allowed to treat anyone who is unwilling to be helped.

With Michael's stubborn refusals, the paramedics could do nothing but leave. He continued to lie on his couch, day in and day out. On the fourth day, he lost consciousness, and Katharine again called paramedics. This time, the unconscious Michael was in no condition to object. But they were too late. In the end, I ruled that Michael's death was not a homicide as had been suspected by the roommate nor natural as deemed by the hospital, but accidental—caused by a fall and muscle damage.

Lack of timely medical care can lead to disaster! Even if you aren't afraid to go to the doctor, it's important to figure out when you need to go. Here are two axioms to follow. Seek medical attention immediately if: (1) you experience any symptom that causes an interruption in your day so severe that you can't go on with what you've planned; (2) you experience any symptom that wakes you up at night and is so bad that you can't sleep through it.

What kind of symptoms might interrupt your day or your sleep? To help identify a serious under-the-radar health problem, I've rounded up the most common covert conditions that warrant a doctor's attention, and they're listed in the table on page 25.

Many of these signs represent a significant medical emergency, and you should head straight to the emergency room. If you're experiencing symptoms such as chest or upper abdominal pain or pressure, dizziness or shortness of breath, uncontrolled bleeding, or severe vomiting, a visit to the ER is a must. Deep cuts or wounds that might require stitches are another "must go" situation. The faster you get treated, the better your prospects for survival and recovery. Lost moments can result in death. The ER, however, should not be used for sniffles and sneezes, earaches, and chronic diseases or routine care you'd normally see your doctor for.

Get Checked

Do you really need a checkup once a year? The answer to this simple question is not without controversy. On one hand, maybe not, says the U.S. Preventive Services Task Force, a government agency that studies the efficacy of medical procedures and tests. On the other hand, many primary care physicians recommend annual physicals.

I come down on the side of *yes*, we do need annual physicals, if for no other reason than to build a relationship with your doctor and talk about preventive health. Research says that people who have good relationships with their doctors are more satisfied with their health care—and get better care.

Your yearly checkup is a great opportunity to get counseling from your doctor about personal health habits. Getting a doctor's help to change bad habits may

DON'T IGNORE THESE SYMPTOMS!

Symptom	What It May Mean
Difficulty breathing, shortness of breath	Obstructive pulmonary disease (asthma or emphysema), bronchitis, heart problems, panic attacks, pneumonia, a blood clot in the lungs (pulmonary embolism), pulmonary fibrosis, anemia, upper airway obstruction, overdose, or collapsed lung
Chest or upper abdominal pain or pressure	Heart attack, tearing of the aorta, pancreatitis, pulmonary embolism, inflammation around the heart, gallbladder attack, ulcers, or pneumonia
Fainting, sudden dizziness or weakness	Heart attack, stroke, abnormal heart rhythm, heart valve abnormalities, or seizures
Changes in vision	Stroke or transient ischemic attack (TIA), bleeding in the inside of the eye, or clotting of the blood vessels of the eye
Confusion or changes in mental status	Infection, head injury, low blood sugar, medication interaction or overdose, meningitis, or encephalitis (inflammation of the brain)
Any sudden or severe headache	Stroke, blood vessel inflammation (vasculitis), meningitis, brain tumor, ruptured aneurysm (weakened blood vessel), brain abscess, uncontrolled high blood pressure, or bleeding on the brain after a head injury

Uncontrolled bleeding	Cancer, leukemia, low platelets, or liver failure
Severe or persistent vomiting or diarrhea	Gastritis (inflammation of the lining of the stomach), gallbladder attack, appendicitis, hepatitis, pancreatitis, obstruction of the bowel, infection in the abdominal cavity, or pregnancy
Coughing blood	Tuberculosis, cancer, pneumonia, bronchitis
Vomiting blood	Inflammation of the esophagus or stomach, ulcers, varices (torn blood vessels at the end of the esophagus), or cancer
Suicidal or homicidal feelings	Depression, mental health problems
Unexplained weight loss	Overactive thyroid (hyperthyroidism), depression, liver disease, cancer, diabetes, tuberculosis, AIDS, or disorders that interfere with how well your body absorbs nutrients (malabsorption disorders)
Unexplained changes in bowel habits	Bacterial or viral infection, parasitic infection, inflammatory bowel disease, colon cancer, or medication side effects
Unusual weakness or fatigue	Heart attack (especially in women or the elderly), heart failure, anemia, low thyroid (hypothyroidism), liver or kidney disease
Loss of consciousness after a fall	Bleeding around the brain (subdural hematoma), especially in people on blood thinners

Thirst and frequent urination	Diabetes mellitus, diabetes insipidus (inability to concentrate urine)
New onset of seizures	Brain tumor, bleeding on or in the brain, or vasculitis (inflammation of the blood vessels in your brain), blood electrolyte abnormalities, stroke, meningitis, or encephalitis
Persistent fever	Tuberculosis, endocarditis (bacterial infection of the heart valves), vasculitis, tumor, lymphoma, lupus, or malaria (if you've traveled to malaria-prone regions of the world), other infections
Trouble swallowing or painful swallowing	Esophageal cancer or throat cancer, infection of the throat or esophagus, neurologic problems, or AIDS
Persistent hoarseness	Throat cancer or other malignancies
Severe, incapacitating back pain	Myeloma, metastatic cancer, leaking aortic aneurysm or torn aorta, epidural abscess (abscess around spinal cord), shingles, or slipped or herniated discs
Hot, tender, or swollen joints	Joint infection, acute arthritis, gout, or vasculitis
Severe diarrhea	Infection due to viruses, bacteria, or parasites, inflammatory bowel disease (Crohn's disease or ulcerative colitis), or AIDS

Is It Heartburn or a Heart Attack?

I call it the "pink stomach syndrome."

At autopsy, the person's stomach is coated with a bright pink paste. This tells me, before I even dissect the heart, that the decedent probably died of a heart attack.

How do I know? Many supposed cases of indigestion are actually a symptom of a heart attack. People are often too willing to assume that "it's just something I ate," and they pop some Pepto-Bismol pills or take the liquid for relief, when they're really having a heart attack. Later, the person is found dead. If there's an autopsy, there will be traces of the antacid in the stomach—hence the pink stomach syndrome.

Yes, heart attacks do sometimes announce themselves with a Fred Sanford moment. "This is the big one, Elizabeth," as Sanford, played by Redd Fox on the 1970s sitcom *Sanford and Son,* used to say as he clutched his chest and gazed heavenward. But the severe crushing pain people imagine when they think of a heart attack is not always present. For 30 percent of people who die from heart disease, indigestion or another seemingly unrelated symptom was their only warning. Passing off sudden or severe indigestion is a recipe for disaster.

The typical pain of a heart attack is squeezing pain in the chest, a feeling of fullness, or pressure that lasts for several minutes. These signs may be accompanied by light-headedness, shortness of breath, sweating, or nausea. The pain may radiate to either shoulder, the back, the arms or the hands, the neck, or the jaw. If you experience any of these symptoms, it's important to call 911 immediately, take an aspirin (unless you have an allergy to aspirin or have been told not to take it by your doctor), and go to the emergency room by ambulance. Don't attempt to drive yourself.

The only way to safely rule out a heart attack is to be seen by a doctor as soon as possible and allow diagnostic tests to be run. The most important thing to remember when dealing with chest discomfort is this: Every moment counts. If your pain is caused by a heart attack, the longer you wait to seek treatment the more severe the damage to your heart could be. Don't fool around with chest pain. Your life could be at stake.

save more lives than often-repeated diagnostic tests. In other words, does your doctor help you quit smoking or simply give you a chest X-ray to see if you've dodged the bullet one more year? Does he or she seem worried that you're eating a bunch of stuff dietitians forbid?

The annual physical is also time to have your cholesterol, blood pressure, and blood sugar tested. Ideally, your total cholesterol level should be less than 200 mg/dl; your HDL (the "good" cholesterol) 35 mg/dl or higher; and your LDL (the "bad" cholesterol) less than 100 mg/dl. Normal blood pressure is 120 over 80, and normal fasting blood sugar is less than 100 mg/dl. Keeping your cholesterol, blood pressure, and blood sugar within healthy ranges through diet, exercise, and sometimes medication will help maximize your longevity.

Your primary care physician can also keep you up-to-date on immunizations and other screening tests you might need, based on your health status, risk factors, and your family history of certain diseases. Adult vaccinations are an often-overlooked component of a preventive program. In the tables on pages 30, 32, and 34, I've listed the screening tests and vaccinations you may need, but always check with your doctor to see which ones apply to you and how often you should have them.

Get the Most Out of Your Next Doctor's Visit

A doctor's appointment is a visit most people dread. Just the thought of putting on one of those gowns that fits like a bib is enough to make you want to cancel your appointment altogether. But don't worry. Instead of dreading a date with

MAJOR SCREENING TESTS FOR WOMEN: WHAT YOU NEED AND WHEN

Screening Test	When
Body mass index (BMI) measurement	Each health-care visit.
Blood cholesterol test	Regularly, starting at age forty (earlier if you have diabetes, high blood pressure, family history of heart disease, or you smoke).
Blood pressure measurement	At least every two years. High blood pressure was traditionally defined as 140/90 or higher, but recent data says that you should try to keep your blood pressure near normal, which is 120/80.
Blood glucose (sugar) test	Starting at age forty-five, every three years.
Colorectal cancer screening	Starting at age fifty, every one to ten years depending on the test used.
Clinical breast exam (CBE)	Starting at age twenty, every three years; yearly after age forty.
Mammography	Starting at age forty, yearly.
Pap test	Starting at age eighteen to twenty, yearly. After age thirty, every one to three years, depending on the test used and past results.
Dental exam	Twice a year. (People with gum disease may be more likely to have a heart attack, stroke, or thickening of the arteries. Oral bacteria

	have been found in arterial plaque and can induce a process that leads to blood clots.)
HIV test	At least once; additional testing is important if you have risk factors.

Source: U.S. Department of Health and Human Services

your doc, you can make it a positive and beneficial experience by preparing for your appointment in advance. This helps your doctor diagnose, prevent, and treat any condition that may be troubling you.

When my doctor-husband goes to the doctor, he brings his written medical history, a list of any medicines he's taking, and other medical information, such as recent test results. He's active in his own health care—as we all should be. So prepare for each and every doctor's appointment.

For starters, write down each medication you're taking, who prescribed it, when it was prescribed, and for what condition. Jot down the strength of the medicine, how much you take, and when. Add to this list any over-the-counter (OTC) drugs you're taking or have taken recently, such as vitamin supplements, antacids, or aspirin products.

Whether going in for a routine examination or for a particular problem, you're sure to have questions. Write them down and have them on hand so you can remember to read them to your doctor.

If you're seeing your doctor for a specific medical problem, provide information about your symptoms. Reporting your symptoms is one of three main ways your doctor figures out what's wrong with you. The other two are the physical examination, in which your doctor looks and feels and listens; and tests, from taking your temperature to doing blood tests to running sophisticated scans. But most of the time, an accurate description of your symptoms will lead your doc to the correct diagnosis, even if he later confirms it with the exam and tests.

MAJOR SCREENING TESTS FOR MEN: WHAT YOU NEED AND WHEN

Screening Test	When
Body mass index (BMI) measurement	Each health-care visit.
Blood cholesterol test	Regularly, starting at age thirty-five (earlier if you have diabetes, high blood pressure, family history of heart disease, or you smoke).
Blood pressure measurement	At least every two years. High blood pressure was traditionally defined as 140/90 or higher, but recent data says that you should try to keep your blood pressure near normal, which is 120/80.
Blood glucose (sugar) test	Starting at age forty-five, every three years.
Colorectal cancer screening	Starting at age fifty, every one to ten years depending on the test used.
Prostate specific antigen (PSA) test and digital rectal exam (DRE)	Starting at age fifty. Ask your doctor about this since testing is controversial.
Abdominal aortic aneurysm	If you're between the ages of sixty-five and seventy-five and have ever smoked (one hundred cigarettes in your lifetime), be screened once for abdominal aortic aneurysm, which is an abnormally large segment of your aorta, the major vessel from the heart.

| Dental exam | Twice a year. (People with gum disease may be more likely to have a heart attack, stroke, or thickening of the arteries. Oral bacteria have been found in arterial plaque and can induce a process that leads to blood clots.) |
| HIV test | At least once; additional testing is important if you have risk factors. |

Source: U.S. Department of Health and Human Services

I once autopsied a woman who went to her doctor and described only one symptom: lower abdominal pain. Not long afterward, she died of meningitis. She had never mentioned any symptoms of meningitis, such as fever, headache, stiff neck, and vomiting, so the doctor treated her abdominal pain. The clues you provide are what guide your physician. In the absence of clues, it's tough for your doctor to get it right. You, the patient, will get much better treatment if you supply the information about what you feel and what you sense in your own body. If you're in pain, for example, be as specific as possible about the type of pain you feel. Is it a dull ache, a throbbing ache, a sharp stabbing pain, or a more generalized discomfort? Where? Do you feel the pain only in one place, or does it occur in different places? List these. Does the pain begin in one spot and then seem to move to another? If so, describe it. Also, write down when the pain occurred and how long you've had it. Some problems can come on without pain, of course, so it's important to report any changes you think are significant. Think about it: Who knows your body better than you? Be honest with your health-care professional.

You can follow a few other simple directions to ensure that your visit will be a productive one. Take notes, or have someone come with you to help you understand and remember the information. If there's anything you don't understand, be sure to ask the doctor to explain or illustrate it. Ask for written instructions, too. When you think you understand, restate what you heard so there is no

VACCINATIONS TO PREVENT DISEASE

Shot	When You Need It
Measles-mumps-rubella (MMR) shot	At least once if you have never had this shot as an adult and were born after 1956 (otherwise you have immunity). There have been recent outbreaks of mumps in the United States, and the potential for measles imported from other countries remains high.
Tetanus-diphtheria (Td) shot	Once every ten years. A new tetanus-diphtheria-whooping cough (pertussis) vaccine, DTaP, should be substituted for one of the tetanus-diptheria boosters before age sixty-five. This vaccine will also help to protect young people with whom you come in contact.
Flu shot	Every year after age fifty or sooner if you have lung, heart, or kidney disease, diabetes, or cancer; you are a health-care worker; or you are infected with HIV. I recommend all adults receive the influenza vaccine annually. Influenza and its complications remains one of our largest and most preventable killers.
Pneumonia shot	Once at age sixty-five for healthy adults. Those with chronic illnesses should receive vaccines earlier and may need repeat doses.

Hepatitis B shot	If you engage in risky sexual behavior, have had any sexually transmitted disease within the last six months, have injected street drugs, work at a job that involves contact with human blood or blood products, or travel to areas where hepatitis B is common. This vaccine, given once as a three-shot series, is now universally given to children.
Shingles vaccination	If you are sixty or older, strongly consider this one-time vaccine since shingles can be a devastating, painful illness.
HPV vaccination (for protection against cervical cancer)	Three shots, given in a series, for girls eleven or older or for women age thirteen to twenty-six who have not been previously vaccinated.

Source: U.S. Department of Health and Human Services

question about its accuracy. If the doctor uses words or terms you don't know, ask for a translation. Virtually all medical lingo can be put into easily understandable language. When you participate in the process and help your doctor figure out what's wrong, you'll get much better health care. It's your body, and you've got to take responsibility for it.

TURN THE TABLES: Know Your Cancer Risk for Better Protection

My grandmother had breast cancer, raising the possibility that this cancer runs in my family. To get a sense of your own cancer risk, find out the types of cancer that occurred in your family and bring this to the attention of your doctor. If your family history puts you at higher risk, you may need to be screened more often.

Can You Trust Your Diagnosis? When to Ask for a Second Opinion

In 2006, a large growth was found in my ovaries. My doctor suspected I had ovarian cancer, which is among the most insidious and deadly of cancers. To say I was terrified is to understate the case. I had just remarried, yet in a heartbeat the rhythm of my new life changed. Mark's first wife had died of ovarian cancer; here he was, possibly facing the disease anew with me. It was a very scary time for both of us. We went about our days, acutely aware that a disease of such proportion would disrupt our lives. All the plans, all the hopes we had for the future were put on hold.

I was referred to an oncologist for a second opinion. I asked him many different questions. He laid out all my options and reaffirmed that I needed surgery to determine whether I had cancer. Had I not liked the options, I wouldn't have hesitated to get even a third opinion.

It's always a good idea to get a second opinion when you're facing surgery, you've been diagnosed with a serious illness, or you're at all uncomfortable with your doctor's recommendations. You want to have confidence in your treatment. Don't be embarrassed or feel that you may insult your doctor if you seek another opinion. Say something like this: "I think I'd like a second opinion, do you mind?" Or, "I value your advice, but I'm thinking about getting a second opinion." Occasionally, a doctor will get angry. If that happens to you—run away, fast! You need a doctor who supports decisions that are in your best interest.

Be sure to get an objective second opinion, too. You need an independent evaluation of your case from a physician who is totally unconnected to your doctor. Also important: Make your medical history available to the doctor providing the second opinion.

As for my situation, after my surgery my doctor called to tell me fabulous news: Further tests had found no cancer. When I heard this, every muscle in my body relaxed. I smiled and cried at the same time. Now I could get on with my life.

If you're living with a fear of doctors, the cost to your health could be high. When problems are discovered early, the prognosis can be very good. Your physician plays a critical role in your overall health, but he can't help you if you refuse to see him. Medicine can be wonderful, but it's useless if you won't avail yourself of its healing power.

LIFE LESSONS: Oral Sex Can Lead to Head and Neck Cancers

For much of my medical career, I was taught that head and neck cancers were caused by smoking, heavy alcohol use, and particularly a combination of the two. Now there's a new culprit on the block: human papillomavirus (HPV), the virus that causes cervical cancer. HPV infections appear to multiply the risk of certain head and neck cancers, particularly those of the tonsils, according to researchers. Studies have found that a certain strain of HPV was present in tumor cells in people's mouths and throats and might have been transmitted through oral sex. Medical experts say the HPV vaccine, which is highly effective against cervical cancer, might also lower the incidence of tumors in the head and neck.

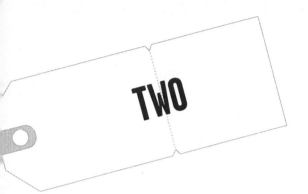

TWO

Deadly Prescriptions

Unhappy Ending

I was worried that I'd have to designate the death of thirty-seven-year-old Nancy Walls as "undetermined" on her death certificate. For months, I tried to figure out what had killed her. I wondered what I had missed, and the case continued to stump me.

Her tragic story began on an evening like any other, when Nancy said good night to her husband, Gordon, age forty. With two kids, and a receptionist's job to make ends meet, she usually tired out early. On this night, she was in bed by 10:30 p.m. Two hours later, Gordon joined her. At about 3 a.m., he heard a noise that sounded like it was emanating from the air conditioner. He banged on the unit a couple of times, before realizing that the strange sound wasn't coming from the air conditioner but from his wife's labored breathing.

In that instant, Gordon flipped on a light. What he saw next jolted him out of bed. Nancy's stomach had risen like an over-yeasted loaf of bread. Shocked and frightened, he dialed 911. Moments later, Nancy stopped breathing, and Gordon started CPR. When paramedics got there, they were able to revive her, but she was barely holding on.

After arriving at the hospital, Nancy was admitted to the intensive care unit. She had already tumbled into a coma. The word "coma," taken from the Greek word for "deep sleep," refers to the deepest sleep imaginable, in which the brain is utterly incapable of responding to its surroundings. Not even thunderous noise or the most piercing pain will awaken the patient.

Eventually, Nancy's brain ceased to function. For the next twenty-four hours, though, her breathing was sustained via an artificial respirator. Doctors ran extensive heart studies, a CAT scan, and a battery of other tests. The diagnostic studies were inconclusive. Only days earlier, Nancy had been a healthy young woman without a thing wrong with her. The next thing her family knew, she was dead. The hospital had no answers as to why this young mother had died. Devastated, Gordon wanted an autopsy. Because of the mysterious circumstances surrounding her death, Nancy Walls became my patient.

During the internal examination, I discovered that the emergency treatments Nancy endured in the hospital would make my task more complicated. A balloon pump used to maintain circulation had lacerated her aorta. Her brain was also extremely soft, a result of prolonged life support, what pathologists call a "respirator brain." I wondered what other bodily witnesses had been silenced forever.

As I pawed gently through her internal organs, looking for clues, I discovered one lead that the hospital had not pursued fully. Her bowel, or colon, was distended with tremendous amounts of liquid and air. I inspected the area further. Although much of the colon appeared healthy, the left portion had died or was barely viable. It was suffused with the telltale dusky bluish hue of organ death. The dead bowel would explain the rapid belly distention the night of her death—which is commonly seen shortly after the bowels are deprived of adequate blood flow and oxygen.

When the colon is deprived of oxygen, it loses its integrity. Bacteria leak into the abdominal cavity and sometimes into the bloodstream. This can cause blood pressure to drop and the heart to eventually stop. Her dead left colon was clearly the initiating event in her downward spiral, but exactly why did Nancy's colon die? No obvious cause revealed itself. What's more, her condition, medically termed ischemic colitis, is a disease that typically befalls the elderly.

In search of more clues, I called Gordon. He was highly emotional—and why wouldn't he be? The woman he loved, the mother of his two children, had died suddenly and no one could tell him why. I asked him to give me time, and he told me to take as much time as I needed. I warned him that there was a chance we would never know what caused her ischemic colitis. I had to prepare him for that.

As my post-autopsy work began, I sent out samples of Nancy's blood and other organs to be analyzed by the toxicology lab. But the results came back negative. Microscopic slides were made of all her organs, which I reviewed, but no reason for the dead bowel was found.

As weeks turned to months, Gordon's concerns turned to desperation. He told me he didn't think he could go on living if he didn't know how or why his wife died.

Just as I was about to designate the case undetermined, I made one final attempt to unravel this mystery. I reexamined what little evidence I had. While looking through the microscope at slices of Nancy's spleen, I stumbled upon some clues. Shaped like a loose fist, the spleen is a honeycomb of little blood vessels through which blood slowly filters. I could see that there were small infarcts (areas of dead tissue caused by clots) in her spleen. Similar clots had likely blocked blood flow to her left bowel, triggering her ischemic colitis. The wall of the bowel had failed to contain the billions of bacteria normally in the gut, and some of this bacteria had entered her bloodstream. Her blood pressure dropped to the point at which her heart stopped beating.

But another key mystery remained. What could have caused the blood clots in someone so young? I dug into the medical literature for an answer. Finally, I found it—in the *Journal of Gastroenterology*. There on the pages of the journal was a nine-year study of women in their thirties who had been stricken with ischemic colitis. Most had one thing in common: They were taking birth control pills.

According to Gordon, six months prior to her death, Nancy decided to use oral contraceptives for the first time in her life. Although the pill is considered one of the world's safest and most effective forms of birth control, each package contains specific warnings. One in particular stood out: Birth control pills may increase the risk of blood clots.

Obviously, only a small percentage of women on the pill ever have blood clots. Most times they aren't deadly. My research, however, led me to believe that Nancy was in that tiny minority. Months into the case, I felt certain that Nancy had died of ischemic colitis from taking birth control pills. I called Gordon with my news.

We decided to meet in person. It was very emotional for me because I knew how much he had suffered. I was about the only person he felt he could talk to about his wife's death. The meeting helped him understand why Nancy was no longer with him. As the facts about her death sank in, Gordon began the process of healing. To friends and family, my findings are often the final chapter in the lives of their lost loved ones—the final word that, though often bittersweet, can offer much-needed peace of mind.

In most cases, medications are lifesavers. They cure infections. They ease pain. They control diseases. They prevent symptoms. But along with their benefits, they have the potential for harm when used incorrectly or paired with substances that cause dangerous interactions. There are also those rare but tragic instances when a perfectly healthy person dies from taking medication exactly as prescribed.

This sounds scary, but there's no need to panic. You shouldn't have any problems as long as you know what you're prescribed, how to take it, and what the possible side effects might be—and are willing to heed the warnings.

How Not to Die from Medication Mishaps

You go to the doctor, get a prescription, have it filled, and take your medicine. What else do you need to know about your medications? Plenty.

No medicine is 100 percent safe for everyone. Useful, familiar, and effective drugs, from acetaminophen for headaches to diuretics to treat high blood pressure, all come with both risks and benefits. Some can produce severe side effects; others pose dangers of allergic reactions, addiction, or toxic interactions if they're mixed with other substances. Any drug you take, including OTC drugs you buy off the pharmacy shelf, can produce what we doctors call an "adverse effect," especially if you take the medicine incorrectly. Adverse effects include side effects, drug-drug interactions, food-drug interactions, and interactions with substances such as alcohol, tobacco, or herbs.

What You Must Know About Adverse Effects

Side Effects

A drug doesn't go to work in a specific spot, but spreads throughout every nook and cranny of your body. Along the way, it can produce untold side effects just about anywhere. Side effects can range from mild and temporary to life-threatening, even when the medications are taken absolutely as directed. A single aspirin tablet, for example, may result in a life-threatening asthma attack in a sensitive person.

Information about side effects comes with prescription medicines and most OTC drugs. Not everyone reacts the same way to a medication. You may experience a reaction to a certain drug, while someone else may have no problems at all. Most side effects depend on your disease state, age, weight, gender, ethnicity, genetics, and overall health. Side effects are usually mild and diminish the longer you take a drug. Sometimes, though, they can be severe—prolonged vomiting, bleeding, vision or hearing changes, and marked fatigue, for example.

> **TURN THE TABLES:** Prevent Skin Cancer
>
> Check labels for warnings about how medicines may increase your body's sensitivity to the sun. Wear a broad-spectrum sunscreen (SPF 30 or higher) that shields you from UVA and UVB rays. Pay attention to label warnings, limit exposure to the sun, and use sunscreen to help prevent skin cancer.

These are warning signs that something is wrong, and you should get in touch with your doctor immediately.

Polypharmacy

Nearly one-third of all adults take five or more different medications. Some patients take up to twenty-five drugs or more a day! Taking multiple drugs is called polypharmacy, and the elderly (age sixty-five and older) are particularly vulnerable to this. The greater the number of drugs you take (prescribed and OTC), the greater the risk of drug-related interactions. For example, an antacid may cause a blood-thinning (anticoagulant) drug to be absorbed too slowly, while aspirin will greatly increase the risk of bleeding with such drugs.

Avoid polypharmacy. Ask your doctor (or doctors) to review your treatment plan at least every three or four months. Drugs you no longer need should be discontinued.

Food-Drug Interactions

Food can interact adversely with drugs, making them work faster or slower, or even preventing them from working at all. Here are some examples: grapefruit juice can increase the blood levels of some drugs, such as sedatives or calcium-channel blockers (used to treat heart disease), increasing the chances of side effects. Calcium in dairy products impairs the absorption of tetracycline and ciprofloxacin, widely used antibiotics. Ask your doctor about food-drug interactions and read the information that accompanies your prescriptions.

Drugs and Alcohol

Many people don't think twice about having a cocktail while on medication. But please know that chronic alcohol use can cause changes in the liver that speed up the metabolism of some drugs, including anticoagulants and drugs used for diabetes. Drugs, many of them lifesaving, become less effective because they do not stay in the body long enough.

Heavy, chronic drinking can also damage the liver so that it's less able to metabolize or process certain drugs. In that case, the drugs stay in the system too long. Acetaminophen, a common OTC pain medication, may be especially dangerous when combined with heavy alcohol use. Both are toxic to the liver and can produce a deadly synergy.

Alcohol depresses the central nervous system (CNS). When taken along with another CNS-depressant drug such as a tranquilizer, alcohol can blunt performance skills, judgment, and alertness. If the mixture includes barbiturates, diazepam (Valium), or propoxyphene (Darvon), the result can be fatal. Drugs and alcohol don't mix! Deaths from combining alcohol and CNS-depressant drugs are almost a daily occurrence in my morgue.

Drugs and Herbs

Nearly one in five people in the United States report using an herb to treat a medical problem or to improve their health. More than half don't disclose this information to their doctors or nurses, according to research. This kind of silent treatment is asking for trouble, especially if you combine certain herbal medicines with prescription drugs.

For example, Saint-John's-wort, a popular mood-lifting herbal remedy, may increase the risk of confusion, nausea, and diarrhea—symptoms of an excess of the neurotransmitter serotonin—when taken with antidepressants such as Prozac. Ginkgo biloba can trigger bleeding if you're taking warfarin, a blood thinner. Yohimbine, an anti-impotence herb, can provoke hypertension when combined with tricyclic antidepressants.

Herbal supplements taken alone can spell trouble, too. Some herbal supplements have been found to be contaminated with selenium, lead, or arsenic, and others have even been "doctored" with drugs such as steroids. Certain herbal supplements such as ginkgo biloba or garlic can affect the success of surgery by decreasing the effectiveness of anesthesia or triggering dangerous complications, such as bleeding or high blood pressure. Always tell your doctor about any herbs you're taking.

Drugs and Smoking

Nicotine and other tobacco products can speed up the metabolism of some drugs. Thus, if you're a smoker, you may need larger-than-normal doses of these drugs. And if you stop smoking, the dosage may have to be changed. All sorts of adverse reactions can occur when smoking is in the picture.

Adverse Drug Effects: Fight the Risk!

Since I graduated from medical school in 1982, so many more drugs have hit the market that it's impossible for any doctor to keep on top of all possible interactions. In 2004, there were nine thousand generic and thirty-three thousand branded drugs in use in the United States alone!

You, the patient, have to do your part to help. Whenever your doctor pulls out a prescription pad, remind him or her of the other drugs, OTC medications, vitamins, and supplements you're taking. Better yet, keep an up-to-date list you can show to your doctor. Also, bring up any drug allergies you have and share if you're being treated for a different condition by another doctor. Let your doctor know if you smoke, use alcohol, or are pregnant or breast-feeding. With this information, she or he can help you minimize the possibility of harmful interactions and make sure that you aren't taking something you don't need. Another way you can reduce the risk of adverse drug effects is to go to reputable websites like www.medscape.com or www.drugs.com. These sites have "interaction checkers," tools that let you to plug in the medicine you're taking to get a list of all the drug's interactions.

Before leaving the doctor's office with your prescription, make sure you can read it. If you can't, your pharmacist might not be able to, either. Also, ask your doctor or nurse what the medicine is for, how often you should take it and for how long, whether you should take it on an empty or full stomach, whether you should avoid certain foods, beverages, or activities while taking it, and what its common and uncommon side effects are. Very important: Ask your doctor what you should do if these side effects do occur. Write this information down.

Unless it's essential, don't use any prescription drug within two years of its approval, either. In the past decade or so, the U.S. Food and Drug Administration (FDA) has yanked a dozen or more medicines off the market for catastrophic adverse effects that were not known when the drugs were first launched. If a relatively small number of studies show that a drug works and is safe, the FDA approves it. But once the drug has been on the market for a couple years and millions of people have used it, infrequent but serious problems may surface.

I remember when the new COX-2 inhibitors debuted as a treatment for arthritic pain. My doctor was singing their praises and gave me a whole bag of free samples to treat some arthritis at the base of my thumb. I refused to take them because they were too new. Ibuprofen and aspirin worked fine for me. Sure enough, some of the widely heralded COX-2 inhibitors were later withdrawn from the market due to an increased risk of heart attack and stroke.

Bugs Versus Drugs

Doctors hear it all the time: "I've got a cold. Give me antibiotics!"

The trouble is, antibiotics fight bacteria. Colds are caused by viruses. Still, patients demand antibiotics for illnesses that don't require them, and physicians often oblige them.

The upshot of this massive antibiotic exposure and overuse is a serious predicament: Dozens of different kinds of bacteria—nicknamed "superbugs"—have developed resistance to one or more antibiotics. As a result, infections that were easily cured by older antibiotics now require expensive, newer drugs. And a few bugs are resistant to almost all antibiotics.

Be smart: Don't take, or ask for, antibiotics unless you really need them.

Unless it's a new cancer drug and you've got the cancer it's designed to treat, stick with what's tried and true, and don't succumb to ads pushing new drugs.

When using any kind of drug, it's important to read the label for instructions. Sometimes medication labels can be hard to understand. For example, if it says four times daily, does that mean taking a dose every six hours around the clock or just during regular waking hours? Anyone can become seriously sick from exceeding a drug's recommended dosage. If you read the label and still have questions, call your doctor, nurse, or pharmacist for help.

OTC Alert: Dietary Supplements

Researchers estimate that approximately 50 percent of adults in the United States use dietary supplements, and 33 percent take multivitamin/multimineral supplements. Many people automatically assume that over-the-counter dietary supplements are safe, but many can have harmful side effects, especially in high doses. Vitamins and minerals can cause problems if taken with some drugs. And many people don't consult their doctors about their supplement regimens. They experiment without the benefit of knowing about possible side effects or interactions.

Dying to Be Young

This issue brings to mind one of the most puzzling and longest-running cases I've ever investigated—the case of forty-nine-year-old Lisa Aarons, who in April 2004 was found dead in her Orlando home early one Monday morning. Nothing suspicious turned up at the scene; it was just a sudden, unexpected death.

Lisa's death was a real mystery to me from the start. From what I learned, this slim, dark-haired beauty seemed so healthy. She exercised every day. She religiously watched her diet and kept her weight around 118 pounds. She didn't drink, smoke, or take drugs. She hadn't mentioned suicide, nor was she depressed. Her husband, Peter, told me that at 2:30, the morning of her death, he was awakened by an odd sound—a gasp. I suspected that the sound may have been Lisa's final breath.

Peter left for work as usual on Monday, thinking his wife was asleep. He didn't know she was already dead.

During the autopsy, an unusual scenario began to take shape. Neither the external nor the internal examination turned up anything that would explain Lisa's death. There was no evidence of an injury, congenital problems, or medical disease. From what I could tell, Lisa should have still been very much alive. Such unexplained, sudden deaths are rare, and the lack of clues bothered me.

I held out hope that the microscopic evaluation and toxicology lab would give me the answers. The laboratory mounted tissue samples from her heart onto nearly thirty slides. Irregularities in heart function can often lead to sudden death. I spent several hours eyeing the slides under the microscope, only to come up short. There were no heart abnormalities, either at autopsy or under the microscope.

Samples of Lisa's bodily fluids and tissues had been sent to toxicology to screen for thousands of substances, including drugs, alcohol, and poisons. But to my surprise, not one suspicious substance turned up that would pinpoint the cause of death.

Still, I did not want to give up on the case until I knew that I had exhausted every possible avenue. I called Peter to see if he could provide any further insights into his wife's untimely death. What I learned was that this was a man very much in love with his wife. Peter felt I was Lisa's last physician, and I felt I owed it to him to help him move through the grieving process. Rather than declare the case undetermined, which was an option, Peter and I set about trying to uncover the truth.

Through a series of phone calls and face-to-face meetings with Peter over many months, startling new revelations came to light. In the days and weeks before her death, Lisa had been experiencing mood swings. Where once she had had a very sweet, even-keeled personality, she was suddenly given to outbursts of irritability. She wasn't sleeping well. I asked Peter about her hair. In photographs, it was thick and full, but it looked thin and patchy at the autopsy. He told me that, yes, her hair was falling out, and she had started wearing a wig.

But it was Peter's next recollection that proved to be the most disturbing of all—a few weeks prior to her death, Lisa had been experiencing heart palpitations.

To me, Lisa's list of assorted and disconnected symptoms pointed to some sort of hormonal imbalance. But Peter insisted that his wife's health was excellent. As he elaborated on her exceedingly healthy lifestyle, he inadvertently revealed a clue that broke the case wide open: Lisa was taking as many as forty vitamin and dietary supplements each day.

At that point, I began to suspect that the supplements might be implicated in her death, just because of the sheer volume she was taking. With Peter's help, my next step was to determine what supplements Lisa was taking and where they came from. We combed through her pill bottles and receipts. We discovered that Lisa was spending more than two hundred dollars a month on supplements, some from foreign countries and banned in the United States. As we scrutinized everything, one supplement stood out: DHEA.

DHEA (short for dehydroepiandrosterone) is a naturally occurring hormone made in the adrenal glands (tiny sacs that sit atop the kidneys) that helps manufacture the sex hormones estrogen and testosterone. Production rises dramatically during puberty but wanes as we age. Supplement manufacturers have promoted DHEA as a cure-all for everything from obesity to heart disease to aging, sometimes on the basis of flimsy scientific evidence. The hype sounds pretty good. I want to look and stay young, too; who doesn't?

But anytime you boost the level of sex hormones in the body, as DHEA does, you risk triggering some pretty strange side effects. It has been suggested by some medical experts that large amounts of DHEA, especially when taken with other dietary supplements, may alter the contractions of the heart, causing it to beat irregularly. A heart arrhythmia like this could be fatal, even the first time it happens.

Lisa was taking seven times the recommended dosage of DHEA every day.

Peter was also using the supplement and had complained of heart palpitations, too. His heart palpitations stopped when he stopped taking DHEA after Lisa's death. I don't think this was a coincidence.

My suspicion that Lisa's death may have been caused by taking excessive doses of DHEA would remain a theory unless I could prove that she had abnormal levels in her system at the time of her death. I asked our toxicology lab to check levels of the hormone in Lisa's blood. Unfortunately, her blood samples had degraded too much to detect any DHEA, even if the hormone was in her system at high levels at the time of her death.

Sometimes in my work, I can't prove things beyond a shadow of a doubt. In this case, I had to read between the lines and go with the preponderance of the circumstantial evidence, which included Lisa's symptoms and the known effects of DHEA. Since DHEA can be an irritant to the heart, megadoses of this hormone, in combination with the other supplements, appeared to have taken their toll on Lisa's body. The night she died, her normal heartbeat became disturbed. As a result, blood wasn't pumped to her tissues. Her body and brain starved of oxygen, Lisa died suddenly. I concluded that Lisa Aarons died of a heart arrhythmia brought on by excessive supplement use.

This case presented one of life's cruel ironies. Here was a woman taking a huge assortment of dietary supplements to help her stay youthful and healthy, but in the end, they cut her life short. We need to be watchful of what we put in our bodies. The body is a beautiful machine. It regulates itself most of the time, particularly with good nutrition from food, and it doesn't need to be pumped full of massive quantities of supplements.

What you may not know is that while many Americans consider supplements as drugs, the law treats them differently. In 1994, Congress passed a law that essentially limits the FDA's ability to regulate dietary supplements—a law that came about after a lot of lobbying by supplement makers. Since then, the FDA has been powerless to judge the safety of supplements before they get on the shelves.

I think it's fine to take a daily multivitamin/multimineral tablet, and perhaps other supplements depending on your doctor's recommendation. With many supplements, however, you don't really know what you're putting in your body, and they might be harmful. The science on supplements is complex and often inadequate. Take calcium, for example. Calcium supplements are known to be helpful and generally safe, yet taking calcium pills may increase the risk of death due to cardiovascular disease in older women. Excessive amounts of vitamins can be toxic. For example, high doses of vitamin E supplements (400 IU a day or greater) increase the risk of bleeding, and too much vitamin A can cause liver damage, hair loss, and neurologic problems. And even fish oil supplements, which reduce the risk of heart attacks in most patients, have been shown in a recent study to increase the risk of sudden death in certain male heart patients by promoting irregular heartbeats.

All therapy, even dietary supplements, has risks and benefits. Always check with your doctor about taking supplements. Popping lots of dietary supplements can never take the place of a healthy diet and is unlikely to significantly extend your life.

Not What the Doctor Ordered

Mistaken Identity

I've handled thousands of cases as a forensic pathologist. Certain deaths never leave my mind because I relate to them on a personal level. One day, when I was the medical examiner in Bexar County, Texas, the body of a ten-year-old boy lay on the stainless steel table before me. Here was a case that would touch me at my core. Normally, I don't get emotionally involved in cases. It's my job to find answers and come up with a cause of death. People are counting on me to keep my emotions out of it. But with this one, I couldn't help thinking that this little boy will never graduate from high school or college, never buy his own car, never fall in love, and never have a family of his own—all the dreams I had for my own ten-year-old son.

As it happened, this boy died of a terrible, tragic error. The story of how he came to be lying in our morgue that day and how the circumstances of his death were discovered teaches some important lessons about how forensic pathologists go about our work.

Determining why he died was difficult at first. He had a history of asthma, and we speculated that perhaps the asthma had killed him. But after doing the autopsy and reviewing the microscopic sections of his lungs, it was clear that his asthma wasn't serious enough to kill him. For the cause of death, we turned to the toxicology laboratory.

The lab reported that there was a high level of methadone in the child's blood, enough to kill him. Methadone is a legal drug for weaning addicts off heroin. It's often used for the management of pain, and its illicit use is a growing problem.

There must be a mistake, we thought. How would a ten-year-old kid get his hands on methadone? It didn't make sense, so we repeated the tests. Again, they came back positive for lethal levels of methadone.

We talked to the boy's mother. Was she on methadone? Was anyone in the family on methadone? Was the kid acting up and given methadone in an attempt to quiet him down? The answers were no, no, and no.

As it turned out, the boy was undergoing treatment for attention deficit disorder (ADD) and taking the standard ADD drug, Ritalin. For several days prior to his death, he had been feeling uncharacteristically groggy and sleepy. Concerned, his mother notified the doctor, who suggested cutting the Ritalin pills in half. She did so, but his lethargy continued up until the time he was found dead in his bed. We ultimately tested those pills and discovered they were not Ritalin at all. They were methadone.

The generic name for Ritalin is methylphenidate—very close alphabetically to methadone. The unthinkable had occurred: a pharmacy error. This case was tragic, and though it was no more tragic than many I handle, the difference was that it hit home, because I was the mother of a boy the same age. My heart went out to this mom, who was doing everything right to help her son but in the end was failed by a sometimes imperfect health-care system. I have never forgotten that case.

Sadly, this is not an isolated occurrence. Pharmacies do slip up. Some slipups, like a misspelled address, for example, won't hurt anyone, but many other errors could cause serious discomfort, harm, or even death. In fact, the Institute of Medicine (IOM) estimates that 1.5 million people are sickened, are injured, or die annually as a result of medication error. The FDA reports that about 10 percent of all medication errors are from drug name confusion, and the World Health Organization (WHO) says that this confusion is an urgent worldwide problem.

Fortunately, most errors are preventable with vigilance on your part. Here are some of the best ways to protect yourself and your family:

- When you pick up your medicine from the pharmacy or are given medicine in the hospital, ask: Is this the medicine that my doctor prescribed? Researchers at the Massachusetts College of Pharmacy and Health Sciences found that 88 percent of medication errors involved the wrong drug or the wrong dose. Compare what you wrote down at your doctor's office with what's dispensed at the pharmacy.

- Watch out for look-alike drug names. Is that Ceftin or Cefzil? Prinivil or Proventil? There have been numerous reports of pharmacists (and doctors) confusing the drugs, with patients requiring hospitalization as a result.

- Find a pharmacy you like and stick with it. A pharmacist who knows you may be more likely to notice something unusual about a prescription. Also, your medication history will be in the computer system, helping to avoid risky drug interactions.

- Discuss your prescription with your pharmacist if possible, especially if it is a new prescription. He or she can tell you about any side effects and interactions with other drugs, plus confirm that you've got the right medicine.

- Know the color and shape of the pills you take regularly. This prevents you from taking the wrong one. Many drugs have their own websites, complete with pictures. Another excellent source of visual information is the *Physicians' Desk Reference,* which is available in many libraries, or at www.pdr.net.

- Examine the actual pills. The name of most brand-name drugs is usually stamped on the tablets. Also, study the bottle's label. If the information doesn't match the doctor's prescription, notify the pharmacist.

- Read the written information that is provided with the prescription. If you don't understand it, ask your pharmacist for clarification.

- Check everything before you leave the pharmacy. Lots of people simply pay and run. Pharmacists have been known to put a properly filled

COMMONLY CONFUSED MEDICATIONS

Adderall—for attention deficit disorder	Inderal—for high blood pressure
Flomax—for an enlarged prostate	Fosamax—for osteoporosis
Lamisil—for fungal infections	Lamictal—for epilepsy
Hydralazine—for high blood pressure	Hydroxyzine—for hives and itching
Norvasc—for high blood pressure	Navane—for psychosis
Paxil—for depression	Plavix—a blood thinner
Prilosec—for acid reflux	Prozac—for depression
Serzone—for depression	Seroquel—for schizophrenia
Zantac—for ulcers	Xanax—for anxiety
Zidovudine—for AIDS	Zovirax—for herpes

bottle in the wrong bag. Or a pharmacy clerk may mistakenly hand you another customer's order. Make sure it's your name on the bag. Then take the bottle out and check the label as well.

- If you feel ill after taking a drug, report your symptoms immediately to your physician. Don't delay.

On the clinical side, medication errors are being reduced through the use of electronic prescriptions, or e-scripts. E-scripts let doctors send prescriptions to pharmacies by e-mail. One Harvard study found that prescription-drug errors declined by half with e-scripts because pharmacists don't have to decipher a doctor's hieroglyphics or type the prescription into their own computers. Another advantage of e-scripts is that when a doctor writes a prescription, the system can flag possible interactions with other drugs you're taking or question unusual dosage levels.

Another approach being advocated to help minimize errors is having the physician indicate the reason for the drug on the prescription. It's rare for two sound- or spelled-alike drugs to have the same action.

Should You Switch to a Generic?

I economize wherever I can, so I like generic drugs because they save me money on prescriptions. The average savings is between 30 and 40 percent but may be as high as 80 percent in some cases. Generic drugs have the same active ingredients as their more expensive brand-name counterparts. For a generic drug to be FDA approved, the drug company must provide sufficient data that its product has the same effect in the body as that of the brand name. Ask your doctor to write out the generic name or to indicate on his prescription that the pharmacist is at liberty to substitute a generic equivalent of a brand-name drug. Keep in mind that when you do switch to a generic drug, it will have a different color and appearance.

These are wonderful innovations to protect us from medication errors. But honestly, it's often the low-tech solutions that will keep you from dying. This means taking a more active role in your health care, understanding your medications, monitoring them, and getting prompt medical attention if you get sick from a drug.

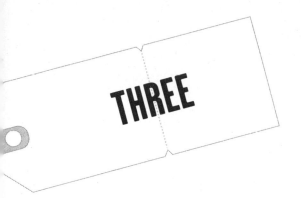

THREE

Code Blue

Fetal Error

I picked up a soup ladle and started bailing blood out of the eighteen-year-old girl's abdominal cavity. I wanted to measure how much blood had drained out of her cardiovascular system. The total amount shocked me: a full two liters, nearly half the blood in her body. What had killed this young girl was clear: She bled to death internally. But why?

The teenager was Isabel Foster, just out of high school, an independent spirit and avid dancer. Isabel had her heart set on studying musical theater when she got to college in the fall. At the time of her death, she was still living at home with her parents—and recovering from one of the most traumatic events of her life: an unplanned pregnancy. A week earlier she had gone to the hospital, complaining of some unusual vaginal bleeding. The hospital staff performed an ultrasound of her uterus. The test failed to show an embryo, but the pregnancy test was positive. The doctor informed Isabel that her bleeding was from an early miscarriage.

Shaken by the experience, Isabel went home. After two more follow-up visits, her ordeal seemed to be over. Then, just a day and a half later, while watching television on the couch, Isabel fell asleep. When her parents tried to wake her up, she didn't respond. Something was terribly wrong. Isabel's father immediately called 911. Paramedics rushed her to the emergency room, but it was too late. Isabel was already dead. She was sent to me to make sense of what had happened.

Isabel's sudden death stunned her parents and filled my mind with questions. Did Isabel die as a result of a complication from the miscarriage? Could the death have been prevented? Miscarriages can occur in up to 20 percent of pregnancies. They're often the body's natural mechanism of aborting an unhealthy baby. While emotionally traumatic, miscarriages usually cause no physical problems. On rare occasions, a life-threatening infection may develop, but this was clearly not what had killed Isabel.

During the internal examination, I paid close attention to what might have triggered Isabel's massive internal bleeding. Often, internal bleeding is caused by an injury to a major organ such as the liver or spleen, or when blood vessels are diseased or torn by broken bones. But in Isabel's case, I suspected the hemorrhage was related to the reported miscarriage.

I also wondered whether Isabel had undergone a follow-up procedure called a D & C—dilation and curettage—and suffered complications as a result of it. In a D & C, the doctor scrapes out the lining of the uterus to remove any retained products of conception. This procedure limits bleeding and reduces the risk of infection. Although a minor procedure, a D & C is still surgery. In up to 10 percent of D & Cs, complications occur, ranging from infection to uterine injury to perforation. Examining this lining can reveal why the miscarriage occurred. Had Isabel had a D & C, her massive blood loss could be from a perforating injury involving a blood vessel. But without full medical records, I couldn't be sure that Isabel had undergone the procedure.

I homed in on Isabel's reproductive organs for clues. Her uterus appeared intact—no perforations from a D & C. Instead, I found the culprit just inches from the uterus: a 1.8-centimeter hole in one of the fallopian tubes. Fallopian tubes are thin conduits that carry a woman's eggs from her ovaries to her uterus. Somehow Isabel's left tube had been torn open. I immediately realized what must have caused the hole in Isabel's fallopian tube—an ectopic pregnancy.

An ectopic pregnancy is a pregnancy that has developed outside the uterus. A healthy pregnancy takes place in the uterus, where there is plenty of room to grow. But in up to one in forty pregnancies, a fertilized egg on its way to the uterus gets stuck in a fallopian tube, either because the tube is too narrow or because of scarring from surgery or a sexually transmitted disease. The embryo implants itself, digging deeper into the tube as it grows, until the walls can no longer sustain the pregnancy and they rupture.

Despite the risk of a fatal rupture, however, ectopic pregnancies don't often end in death. That's because doctors can typically remove the embryo surgically to keep the fallopian tube from bursting. But the hospital never diagnosed Isabel's ectopic pregnancy. Instead, they treated her as if she had had a normal uterine pregnancy and miscarriage.

Isabel was not killed by a complication from a miscarriage, because she never had one. She never had a D & C, either, the follow-up procedure that would have warned doctors of her ectopic pregnancy. Had she been diagnosed properly, she'd be alive. Suddenly, an explosive question arose in my mind: How could the hospital have made such an egregious error?

Isabel's parents never brought suit against the doctor or the hospital, but for me, the bottom line was clear. If you're properly diagnosed prior to a fallopian tube breaking open, there's no reason to die from this. It is treatable. I don't understand how this happened in this day and age. It's truly not my job to place blame, but in this case, Isabel fell through the cracks of the medical establishment. I wish someone had properly diagnosed this young girl. An untimely death is always devastating to the survivors, but there's an added poignancy when a death is avoidable.

Seeing people like Isabel Foster who die suddenly and unexpectedly keeps me humble, thankful I'm alive, and wiser when I observe the many things I can do to decrease my chances of dying prematurely. Cases like hers also make me grateful for the autopsy.

Even in today's high-tech medical world, the low-tech autopsy—not the glitzy forensic autopsy glorified on television, but the routine autopsy done on patients in morgues—provides a uniquely valuable means of quality control and knowledge. It exposes mistakes and bad habits, evaluates diagnostic and treatment procedures, and even detects new diseases. I think it may be the most powerful tool in the history of medicine, responsible for most of our knowledge of anatomy and disease, and it remains vital for advancing medicine.

Autopsies can also keep medical mistakes from being repeated. As the case of Isabel Foster shows, doctors and hospitals do miss things. But without autopsies, they don't know when they've missed something fatal and so may miss it again. They also miss the chance to learn from their mistakes, and their mistakes might get buried forever.

How Not to Die in the Hospital

The truth is, whether it's for treatment or surgery, most people sail in and out of hospitals and clinics with no problems. But there are still risks, and the hospital can be a dangerous place. According to an Institute of Medicine (IOM) report, a staggering forty-four thousand to ninety-eight thousand Americans die each year as a result of medical errors—wrong diagnoses, inappropriate treatments, preventable infections, technical glitches, and the like—in hospitals alone. That's more people than die in car accidents, of breast cancer, or of AIDS. Such mistakes aren't always single glitches. More often than not, they're system or institutional failures such as breakdowns in communication. Usually a domino effect begins at one point and continues to build to the point of injury or death.

To make matters worse, there isn't just one doctor taking care of you in the hospital; sometimes, it's several—not uncommon, especially if you're critically ill. God love them, they're doing everything in their power to help you, but sometimes it seems that it's no one's job to give you a clear picture of what's happening. Sometimes you don't even know your doctors' names while you're in the hospital. And often, your primary care doctor does not follow your progress in the hospital.

With all the things that can potentially go wrong in a hospital, it can make you feel helpless and out of control. From my experience, one of the best things you can do to protect your health in the hospital is to do your due diligence whenever you have any kind of scheduled surgery or procedure. Don't be passive when you check into a hospital. Take an active role in your care and treatment to cut down on some of the risks. Here's a look at how.

Find Hospitals You Can Trust

Even if you belong to a managed health-care plan, you probably have a choice between at least a couple of hospitals in your area. If so, choose one at which many patients have the procedure or surgery you need. Studies tell us that patients tend to have better results when they are treated in hospitals that have a great deal of experience with their condition. Frequent practice often makes for fewer mistakes.

How can you find out this information? For starters, do an accreditation check. Find out whether each has met the standards for accreditation set by the Joint Commission, which accredits and certifies health-care organizations. Visit www.jointcommission.org or call (630) 792-5000.

If you need a particular procedure, call each hospital and ask how often the hospital performs that procedure. If the hospitals in your area don't keep track, call the state health department and ask if the department or any other agency has this information. The same goes for a surgeon. If this information isn't available, ask the surgeons you're considering how often they perform the procedure each year, how many times they've done it in their career, and what their infection rate is.

Mention Allergies to Everyone

Fatal Reaction

Adrienne Michaels, a fifty-six-year-old woman from Kissimmee, Florida, slipped in the shower and suffered a compression fracture in her spine. Compression fractures are actually collapsed vertebra and are extremely debilitating. One of the promising ways to fix this type of fracture is through a procedure called vertebroplasty, in which a cement (made of acrylic) is injected into the crushed vertebra to stabilize it. Adrienne was treated in this way.

Yet soon after this seemingly routine procedure, Adrienne inexplicably died. To figure out why, I had to take into account her symptoms prior to her death, along with what I found at autopsy. In Adrienne's case, observers reported that she had complained of having a lump in her throat. Moments later, she was gasping for air and lost consciousness. Within minutes, Adrienne suffered respiratory arrest, and her heart stopped.

What she was experiencing is known as anaphylaxis, a violent misguided systemic attack by the body's immune system, usually in response to something eaten or injected. It's so overwhelming that it can leave virtually every body system in a state of collapse, and so ferocious that a patient can be dead in minutes despite the best medical treatment. Other symptoms that signal the onset of this reaction include itching and flushing, hives, nausea, and vomiting. Adrienne's symptoms, combined with what I found at autopsy, told the story: cardiac arrest due to an allergic reaction to the acrylic cement.

Allergies and reactions can be a serious, even life-threatening, problem, and some are unknown, as this case shows. Your doctor and nurse will probably ask, but make sure you inform them about your allergies to drugs or other chemicals, such as antibiotics, contrast dye, aspirin, or latex, when you're admitted to the hospital. Don't hold anything back.

What You Can Catch in the Hospital

Hospitals around the country are loaded with the latest medical equipment and technology to help you get well. Unfortunately, they're also loaded with nasty bugs—and not the kind that live in your yard or garden, either. I'm talking about bacteria and viruses that can make you deathly ill. I don't think there's any place where you're more likely to get sick than a hospital. According to the Centers for Disease Control and Prevention (CDC), there are 1.7 million health-care-associated infections every year, and that's cause for alarm if you become a hospital patient.

Dead on Arrival

Not long ago, I autopsied a thirty-four-year-old businessman from Chicago named Hunter Burke, who was attending a convention in Orlando. He fell ill with severe back pain and called his doctor back home for advice. All the doctor did was advise him to take some ibuprofen or acetaminophen. He followed those orders but to no avail. Hunter got so ill that he called 911. He arrested on the way to the hospital and was dead on arrival.

His death mystified everyone, including me. Here was a young, muscular guy—a rugby player to boot—who had died suddenly for no apparent reason. The day his body came to my morgue was uncharacteristically slow, so I picked up the phone and called his wife myself to get some history on him, although my investigator usually does this for me. His wife confirmed that he had been in perfect health, but something odd had happened several weeks ago. He had been diagnosed with a spider bite that had since cleared up, supposedly with the help of antibiotics. The bite was on his back, and he had been complaining of back pain ever since.

So here was Hunter Burke lying on the stainless steel slab in my morgue. Believe it or not, some people look good, even when they're dead; others can look terrible, as if they had been profoundly ill, and Hunter was one of these. His skin was diffusely mottled, unlike the typical purple discoloration known as lividity, in which the red blood cells settle according to gravity. There was also some dark brown material in his mouth that looked like coffee grounds, which, at the risk of slipping into highly technical medical terminology, we doctors call "coffee-ground vomitus." It's often a sign of gastrointestinal bleeding.

As I began the autopsy, I mentally put together some preliminary theories for Hunter's case. Back pain can point to any number of problems, such as an aortic aneurysm or kidney disease. Or maybe he had a delayed rupture of the spleen from a blow while playing rugby. The spleen lies close to the surface of the body, and a hard blow from something like contact sports is more likely to seriously injure this mushy organ than any other abdominal organ. This case was like a can in your cupboard that has no label. You can shake it a little, or look at its size, but you won't know the contents until you open it up.

So that's what I did. Most of his internal organs looked fine, with the exception of his lungs. There I saw the first ripple of trouble. His lungs appeared infected. I swabbed his lungs and collected a sample of his blood so the microbiology lab could culture and identify what, if any, infectious agent was growing in his tissue. I took tissue samples to look at under my microscope.

Then I removed his bowels, so that I could get a better look at the retroperitoneum, the anatomical space behind the abdominal cavity. There I also found a terrible infection. It had caused a pus-filled abscess in the psoas muscle, which runs from the lower abdomen down the thigh. Pus was oozing out everywhere. All of this suggested a severe infection.

I took samples of the muscle tissue, as well. I had a hunch about what kind of infection this was, since 80 percent of all infections that attack the psoas muscle are of one type, but I would wait for the microbiologists to work up blood and tissue cultures.

Back in my office, I placed the slides under the microscope, twisted the knob to bring things into focus, and scanned across the cellular landscape. What I saw confirmed what I suspected from the autopsy. His muscle tissue was necrotic (or dying), inflamed, and filled with infection-fighting white blood cells. Infection had been swarming through Hunter Burke. But it was the shape of the bacteria that confirmed the cause of the infection. They were clumped together like tiny clusters of grapes—proof of a staph infection (the Greek word "staphylē" means "bunch of grapes"). A few days later, the cultures came back positive for staph, but not just any kind of staph.

MRSA: A Superstrong Bug

Although Hunter Burke didn't know it at the time, the red spot on his back, which he and his doctor thought was a spider bite, was the first sign that his body was infected with a potentially dangerous type of bacteria known as MRSA (methicillin-resistant *Staphylococcus aureus*), a strain of staph that has built-in defenses against many of the antibiotic medicines that exist today. As a result, MRSA (commonly pronounced MUR-suh) infections are difficult to treat. Once it got in his bloodstream and multiplied, Hunter developed severe sepsis. As a result, his blood pressure bottomed out, his heart failed, and he died.

MRSA, first seen in hospitals and nursing homes, has turned up in communities. You can catch it by direct physical contact and, rarely, through airborne exposure. You can pick it up by touching towels, sheets, clothing, bandages, and other items that have been contaminated by a person with the infection. At first the infection is the size of a pimple and is often misdiagnosed as a spider bite. It may remain localized as nothing more than a nuisance infection or turn into a monster, spreading rapidly and turning deadly.

I suspected that Hunter Burke got this infection from another rugby player, since MRSA tends to strike people who are in close physical contact, such as members of sports teams, military recruits, children in day-care centers, patients in hospitals and nursing homes, and prisoners in jails. Once the MRSA had caused the skin infection, it likely slipped briefly into his bloodstream and set up shop in his psoas muscle, a muscle that might have been strained on the rugby field and was therefore vulnerable. When a tissue is damaged, it's a standing invitation to staph. After festering in the psoas muscle and creating an abscess, the staph spilled into his bloodstream with alarming speed, outstripping his defenses and killing him. Scary stories aside, there are ways to prevent both community- and hospital-acquired MRSA.

The best protection against MRSA or any hospital-acquired infection is simple hygiene: hand washing. Sometimes the amount of bacteria under one fingernail is more than on the rest of the hand. Fortunately, in an age when antibiotics are becoming less effective, hand washing remains a remarkably useful defense against the spread of infection. Don't let people touch you in the hospital until you've seen them wash their hands. That goes for *everyone*—including doctors and nurses.

Several years ago, I rushed my son Eric to the ER for stitches after he hit his mouth and knocked two teeth out while playing basketball. In the examination area were three people: one coughing, one with a thermometer in her mouth, and the other with a gash in his leg. As we walked in, the nurse had just taken the thermometer out of one person's mouth, started listening to the lungs of the cougher, and was checking the other guy's wound. Then, she started to look at Eric's injuries, but I wouldn't let her get near him. She had never washed her hands between patients, and that was disgusting! We walked out as fast as we could and went elsewhere for treatment.

While in the hospital, ask all health-care workers who have direct contact with you to wash their hands—even before they put on protective gloves. If

---

TURN THE TABLES: Watch Out for Doctors' Ties

Ties dangle, making contact with various objects, and are regularly handled by their wearers. That's a problem. Ties become colonized with bacteria that could cause disease, and they are rarely washed—which is why my husband never wears a tie during his hospital rounds.

someone's hands are unclean when they put on gloves, the gloves might become contaminated.

Gels are faster to use than soap and water, and they generally do a great job killing bacteria. And gel dispensers are conveniently located, usually inside your room and outside your hospital door. Given the enormous problems hospitals around the world are having with infections, there's no excuse for health-care workers not to practice optimal hand hygiene.

Clostridium difficile: A Bug Behaving Badly

Clostridium difficile is a nasty bug that sometimes inflames the colon after patients are given antibiotics. Even some healthy people (about 2 percent) harbor *Clostridium* among the billions of bacteria in the colon, but most acquire it during a hospital stay. It's usually harmless until antibiotic therapy indiscriminately knocks off the normal bacteria in the gut, while sparing *Clostridium*. The *Clostridium* bacteria then spring to action, proliferating rapidly and producing toxins that attack the colon. The result is diarrhea, inflammation of the colon lining (colitis), and sometimes death. Doctors can treat most cases by stopping the offending antibiotic and prescribing antibiotics that target *Clostridium*. Some patients, however, require emergency removal of their entire colons as a last-ditch effort to save their lives. You can become initially infected if you touch items or surfaces that are contaminated with microscopic amounts of *Clostridium* spores from feces and then touch your mouth or mucous membranes. Health-care workers can spread the bacteria to other patients or contaminate surfaces through hand contact.

Unfortunately, there's a new, highly virulent strain of *Clostridium* on the block that produces much more toxin than its predecessors and is highly lethal. This dangerous form makes it even more urgent that people with *Clostridium,* or people caring for them, thoroughly wash their hands with soap and water after any possible contact with the infected material to avoid spreading the germ or becoming infected themselves. Equally important, doctors and patients must work together to use antibiotics more carefully—a good deal more judiciously than we do now—and reserve them for situations in which they're truly necessary.

To help ward off *Clostridium,* some docs are dosing their patients with probiotic supplements after a round of antibiotics. Probiotics are dietary supplements or foods such as yogurt that contain beneficial, or "good," bacteria or yeasts normally found in your body. These microorganisms may help protect against harmful bacteria by maintaining a robust bacterial population.

Stand Up to Pneumonia: Derailed

Pneumonia is another common hospital-acquired infection, and it can be quite serious. This was the case with seventy-two-year-old Barry Miller, one of my wards when I worked in Texas. While traveling by rail from North Dakota to New Mexico, Barry somehow fell from a train going eighty miles per hour and sustained a head injury but no other significant external or internal injuries. Authorities helicoptered him to a hospital in San Antonio. Barry remained in critical condition and was placed on a ventilator because he was unable to breathe on his own. Eventually, in a procedure known as a tracheostomy, doctors slid a breathing tube down his throat and into the windpipe, or trachea, so that more oxygen could be delivered to his lungs through the ventilator. Despite aggressive and appropriate care in the ICU, he never regained consciousness. After two weeks in the hospital, Barry Miller died.

While performing the internal examination, I discovered that Barry's lungs were full of fluid and pus. This told me that Barry had contracted pneumonia, a significant infection of the lungs. People on ventilators are at high risk for lung infections, because the breathing tube bypasses the normal defenses of the respiratory tract and harbors bacteria and other microorganisms. Up to 25 percent of patients placed on a ventilator develop ventilator-associated pneumonia; up to 50 percent of them may die as a result. His infection wasn't just severe; it's ultimately what killed him.

As to why Barry fell off the train, I concluded by the end of the autopsy that he had suffered a major heart attack. This set off a deadly chain of events. He probably experienced some shortness of breath, went out to get some air, and collapsed and tumbled off the train. He was hospitalized, placed on a ventilator, and caught pneumonia.

Although ventilator-associated pneumonia like Barry's is the most frequent and deadly type, anyone who is hospitalized can develop pneumonia—for several reasons. During recovery from surgery or any other treatment, you might naturally take shallow breaths, since you're on your back and breathing deeply may be painful. After surgery, your lung tissue might partially collapse—a condition called atelectasis—which further increases the risk of pneumonia. Most hospitalized patients undergo a change in the type of bacteria living in the mouth and throat. These new bacteria are adept at causing infection. All of these factors can make it easier for bugs that cause pneumonia to gain a foothold.

So what are some ways to minimize this hospital risk? Deep breathing is one, and hospital staff should give you a device called an incentive spirometer. You blow into it several times every day to strengthen your lung capacity. As soon as you are able, get out of bed and walk around the hospital floor with assistance. Do this several times a day. Becoming mobile as soon as you can prevents atelectasis. If needed, a respiratory therapist will give you breathing exercises that can make a big difference to the health of your lungs. And, as always, hand washing is critical.

Bladder Blues

Urinary tract infections are actually the most common type of infection originating in a hospital. Bacteria can slip into patients via urinary catheters—and these infections can be dismayingly tenacious.

Urinary catheters also limit your mobility and are sometimes jokingly referred to as a "one-point restraint." Being tethered to a urinary catheter, however, is no laughing matter, since immobility while you're hospitalized increases your risk of blood clots, pneumonia, and muscle loss.

While urinary catheters are sometimes necessary, the longer the catheter remains in place, the more likely you are to get an infection or other complication. It's often possible to avoid the catheter and a resultant urinary tract infection by using diapers or a bedpan instead.

An Infection No One Tells You About

While in the hospital, you may need frequent intravenous (IV) medications, blood transfusions, fluid replacement, and/or nutrition given through a central venous catheter (or "central line") placed into one of your major veins. It may stay in place for days or even months, depending on the type of line.

Central lines are essential to providing care during hospitalization, but they can get contaminated when bacteria grow in or around the line and spread to the bloodstream. To prevent these infections, hospital personnel have procedures in place, such as hand washing, changing the bandages around the catheters, and making sure that no catheter remains in a vein longer than needed.

You can help, too. Make sure the hospital staff washes their hands before and after working with your line. Don't be afraid to remind them. Find out how your skin will be cleaned when the line goes in, and what steps are being taken to lower the risk of infection. Avoid contaminating yourself; don't touch your IV catheter site or other tubes. Once your medication and fluid needs can be managed using smaller peripheral IVs in your arms, the central line should come out.

Anesthesia: How to Stay Out of Harm's Way

Like a lot of patients, I find the prospect of anesthesia the most frightening aspect of a hospital experience. It's the loss of awareness and control that bothers me the most. Being put to sleep by general anesthesia is like getting on an airplane: You temporarily place your life in the hands of what you hope is an experienced person.

These days, though, anesthesia is really quite safe, thanks to the many advances in anesthesiology, including the hundreds of new and safer anesthetics now in use. Anesthesiologists monitor their patients closely, too. There's plenty of quality control before, during, and after a patient is put under—quality control of such high standards that it's considered a model for improving patient safety in all areas of health care.

Though the risk of complications is low, take precautions nonetheless. Ask to meet with your anesthesiologist to discuss your options. Some procedures require only a local or regional anesthetic, while others will need a full general anesthetic. Go over the benefits and risks of each one.

Although rare, some people are allergic to certain anesthetics. Let your doctor know if any of your family members has ever had a bad reaction to anesthesia. If you suspect you might be at risk, you can have testing done before the surgery. Make sure your doctors know all the medications you're taking, including over-the-counter drugs or supplements. Also, let your doctor know if you drink heavily (more than a few drinks on most days of the week). For heavy drinkers, postoperative alcohol withdrawal can be life-threatening.

One more tip: If you smoke, quit or stop smoking two weeks in advance of surgery. This helps your lungs adapt better to the effects of anesthesia.

What You Must Know Before Going Under the Knife

There's a lot that can go right with surgery, but a lot that can go wrong, too. One case, memorable to me because the woman looked to have been in great health, involved eighty-four-year-old retiree Sandra Collins. Typically, when the deceased is over sixty-five and there's no sign of trauma, no suspicious circumstances, and the scene of death is undisturbed, I order a toxicology test and leave it at that. No full autopsy. But Sandra had a large suspicious bump on the back of her head. She had been found dead at the bottom of a flight of stairs outside her apartment building.

As I looked her over, her body seemed more suited to climbing stairs than lying lifeless at the bottom of them. She was in good shape and obviously took excellent care of herself. Her friends and family told us she was full of life for her age. In fact, Sandra told her friends that she planned to live to age 104, and they believed her. To think that she died of natural causes just didn't sit right with me. I had to figure out what caused that bump on her head. Was she beaten or did she fall?

After I opened her skull, I found evidence of a traumatic brain injury. First of all, she had a subdural hematoma, an accumulation of blood that occurs when blood from a torn vessel collects between the brain and the skull. Second, her skull was fractured. The injury killed her, but what caused the blow?

The injury itself gave me the answer. Inside Sandra's skull, directly under the fracture site on the right side of the back of the head, I saw only a small bruise on her brain. But there was a large bruise on the front left side of her brain opposite the fracture. When there is bruising on the side opposite to where the head is impacted, this is known as a contrecoup injury. It forms when the brain is slapped hard against the far side of the skull, opposite from where the impact occurred. This type of injury told me that Sandra had died because her head smacked against something, not because something smacked against her head. A blow to the skull from an assailant would have produced a much different injury pattern. Sandra's injury was consistent with a fall. She fell down a flight of steps and suffered a fatal head injury.

But I didn't consider the case closed. There was still one question left: Why did Sandra Collins fall? I reached out to Sandra's friends and loved ones to probe for clues. The first person I talked to was Elizabeth, one of Sandra's closest friends. As Elizabeth shared information from Sandra's life, she revealed a surprising detail about the retiree's last days. It was the missing link, and it wasn't in her medical records. Sandra had had some type of laser procedure to correct her vision. The surgery hadn't gone well, leaving Sandra nearly blind.

The rest of the puzzle pieces fell into place easily. The night Sandra died, she left her second-floor apartment, and, with her poor eyesight, she lost her footing and fell back, striking the back right side of her head against the step. Inside her head, Sandra's brain whipped forward, slapping against the front of her skull. This slap created the fatal contrecoup injury.

For most people, laser eye surgery dramatically improves nearsightedness, farsightedness, and astigmatism. Yet for a few unlucky others, like Sandra, it worsens their vision—forever.

All surgery carries risks, even some of the most common and routine procedures you hear about every day. Discuss your risks, alternatives, and prognosis with your doctor—and take these steps to lessen the chance of a surgical error and avoid complications from surgery:

- Understand what the risks are and how they might be minimized.
- Make sure you, your doctor, and your surgeon are clear on exactly what will be done.
- Have your doctor sign his or her initials directly on the site to be operated on prior to the surgery. You'll be less likely to make "Doctor Removes Wrong Kidney" headlines.
- When a nurse comes to give you medicine, ask what it is and why you need it. Make sure the nurse checks your ID bracelet against the name on the prescription. Medication errors are common in hospitals.
- Ask a family member or friend to be with you and be your advocate, should you not be able to speak up for yourself.
- Speak up if you have questions or concerns. You have a right to question anyone who is involved in your care.
- To minimize the risk of surgical wound infections (which account for about 15 percent of all of hospital infections) after surgery, pay close attention to the surgeons' directions regarding wound care. Doctors also do

their part to prevent infections, including meticulous hand washing, wearing gloves and gowns, preparing the skin preoperatively, and prescribing antibiotics to stave off infections. Some particularly infection-prone procedures, like joint replacement, may be performed in specially designed sterile rooms or with the surgical team dressed in "space suits."

- Uncontrolled bleeding after surgery can be another serious complication. Fortunately, though, bleeding after surgery is not as much of a problem as it once was due to improved surgical techniques. Even so, there are ways to lower your risks further. Make sure your doctor knows every medication—including vitamins, supplements, or herbs—that you use. Common medicines—like the painkillers aspirin and ibuprofen—can thin your blood, increasing the risk of bleeding. So can vitamin E, garlic, ginkgo biloba, and many other supplements. Your doctor will probably instruct you to stop taking any medicine or supplement that might have this effect a week or two before surgery.

- When you're being discharged from the hospital, ask your surgeon to explain the treatment plan you will use at home, and what aftercare precautions you should take, from learning about your medicines to when you can resume your normal activities. Get written instructions on how to care for yourself after discharge. Review what's in writing, and make sure you understand it.

Don't Just Sit There: Prevent Deadly Clots

When you're in the hospital, another significant risk is DVT, or deep vein thrombosis. It is a blood clot that develops in the legs or pelvis when the venous circulation (the blood flowing back to the heart) has become sluggish. It can happen during long airplane flights, but the greatest danger is after surgery. DVT, which can be detected by ultrasound and blood tests, becomes life-threatening when part of the clot in the leg or pelvis breaks away and travels into the arteries of the lungs, where it lowers blood oxygen levels. If large enough, the clot can reduce or stop the heart's output. This complication, called a pulmonary embolism, can cause instantaneous death.

Surgery boosts your risks of DVT—for a couple of reasons. Being immobilized in bed impedes your venous circulation, and blood is more likely to pool and clot in your legs. The trauma of surgery itself also increases the blood's clotting tendency.

Fortunately, careful use of blood thinners and mechanical leg compression devices ("squeezers") in the hospital can slash the risk of DVT without increasing your risk of bleeding. So you should always ask whether you'll be getting preventive treatment. All hospitals provide this treatment, but occasional slipups can leave an immobilized or postoperative patient without protection.

Another method of lowering the risk of DVT is something you can do on your own in the hospital. Stay as mobile as you can before and after surgery. Walk around as soon as possible, to keep the blood moving in your veins and prevent it from collecting in any one place. If appropriate, wear elastic surgical stockings. They press on the veins to keep blood circulating.

Beware: Fatal Footing

Falls in the hospital are a big risk for injury and death—which is why you'll probably be assessed for the risk of falling after being admitted. Your risk goes up based on the medications you're taking. Sedatives, narcotics, or anesthetics, for example, can make you a fall risk, and you'll probably be put on the hospital's fall-protection watch. Laxatives and diuretics have also been linked to increased fall risk. If you're taking several drugs at once, you're considered at the highest risk for falls.

But you can protect yourself. Make sure the nurse call light is within easy reach, and that your bed rails are in place. See that your room gets cleaned in a timely manner to prevent tripping hazards. Wear nonskid slippers when walking around your room. If you're incontinent, have the hospital provide a bedside commode.

Can You Trust Your Lab Results?

You probably assume your doctor will read your test results correctly. Every year, billions of laboratory tests are performed in the United States—at hospitals, commercial sites, and in doctors' offices. With the vast majority of procedures, there's no problem: Results are accurate and are correctly conveyed to doctor and patient. But technicians and doctors do make mistakes in performing and interpreting lab results. Because of the sheer volume of testing and the inherent margin of human error, no lab test can be guaranteed error free. Sometimes an error can have far-reaching implications.

This is precisely what happened to Richard Taylor, a twenty-nine-year-old store clerk and soccer enthusiast living in southwest San Antonio. Known as a charismatic mentor to local teens, Richard promoted the establishment of soccer fields in his community so that kids would have more places to play the popular sport.

One night after watching TV, Richard complained of chest pains. An hour later, he walked into a San Antonio hospital. While alone and waiting for treatment in a triage room, he suffered a seizure and collapsed on the floor. After Richard was rushed to the ICU, doctors discovered that he had sustained a heart attack. Because he was so young and seemingly healthy, the hospital and his family were stunned. On the heels of this news came another shock: Hospital tests on Richard's urine revealed a dangerous stimulant—amphetamine. Amphetamine—commonly called speed—and its sister drug, methamphetamine, are highly addictive stimulants that traumatize the central nervous system. Amphetamines do have a legitimate role in the treatment of certain medical conditions, but Richard had never been prescribed this drug. When abused, amphetamines can trigger seizures and heart attack.

After a week in a coma, Richard passed away. On his death certificate, the hospital wrote "a heart attack due to amphetamine use." His mother protested. She claimed that her son did not do drugs, and she was adamant about it. With the stigma of a drug-related death hanging over her son's memory, Richard's mother wanted her son's name cleared. Richard's body was transferred to my office, where determining who was right—doctors or the young man's grieving mother—would be up to me.

To begin, I conducted a thorough external exam, searching for any evidence that might indicate drug use, such as fresh drug tracks, tiny bruises, or skin ulcers on the arms and feet. I found nothing. However, he might have taken the drug orally.

Next, I had to look inside the body where other signs of drug use might have left some clues. I inspected each of Richard's organs and took samples of bodily fluids. I was particularly interested in examining his heart. Amphetamines can elevate blood pressure to dangerous levels, leading to an enlarged, thickened heart. What I found was a seriously damaged organ. His heart had a massively enlarged left ventricle caused by severe high blood pressure.

Next, I cut open his coronary arteries, the vessels that supply blood to the heart. I discovered a clot in a severely narrowed coronary artery (atherosclerosis). This clot caused his fatal heart attack. This discovery of severe atherosclerosis established the diagnosis of long-standing coronary artery disease. But was it acute amphetamine use that triggered this clot and thus his heart attack and death?

To solve the riddle, we had to locate the original, week-old urine sample taken at the hospital and have it rechecked for amphetamine using a more sophisticated test. I also called Richard's mom to find out more about his medical history. What I learned corresponded to the conditions found at autopsy. His mother told me that they had a family history of young people suffering heart attacks. What's more, Richard had complained to his mother of chest pains, and she'd urged him to seek medical care. She was unyielding in her position that he had never used amphetamines.

When the urine test results came back, they were negative for amphetamines. Richard's mom was right all along.

Hospital screens sometimes cannot distinguish between the stimulants in some cold medicines and amphetamines. Hospital staff may have made a hurried assumption in an emergency. Richard's mother was forced to accept the loss of her son, but she could not accept the hospital's explanation. She was grateful that our findings confirmed what she knew in her heart all along.

While many lab errors may be out of your control, there are steps you can take to increase the chances of accurate results. If you can see the test tube, double-check that your name is on it. If you're in the hospital, make sure your wristband is accurate, so that your test isn't mixed up with someone else's. Let your doctor know about any medicines, supplements, or foods you've recently taken or eaten; some may skew test results. If the result of the test is a surprise, ask your doctor: "Did you expect this? Do you think this is what I have?" If the answers are no, ask that your test be repeated. Get a copy of all your lab results and reports. You have the right to these, and they may be valuable later.

Don't Stay Long

Though insurance companies frown on lengthy hospital stays, your doctor has the last word on when you'll be discharged from the hospital. He or she knows that it's best to get out as fast as you can. The longer you're in the hospital, the higher your risk of complications such as infection, bedsores, or blood clots. Do everything your health-care team asks, so you'll be able to leave quickly. In many cases, it's better to continue your recovery at home, anyway, away from the hum and beep of machines, the clatter of the food trolley, and the loud conversations between nurses passing one another in the halls.

Modern medical care is wondrous, but it's complex. The things that can go wrong in a hospital are almost innumerable. But that doesn't make them right or acceptable. Health care, instead of helping you, might cause needless harm or, worse yet, kill you. That's why I believe so strongly that our health-care system needs to be dramatically improved. Until this happens, you must do what you can to ensure that your hospital stay puts you on the path to recovery—and not to the morgue.

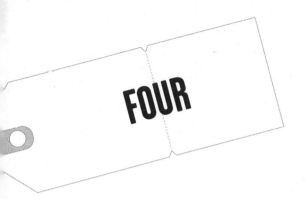

FOUR

Highway to the Morgue

Collision with Death

Shannon Johnson lay on her hospital bed, perfectly still, day in and day out. Nurses and doctors came and went, pricked her with hypodermic needles, asked her questions, and flexed her limbs as machines gurgled, hummed, and buzzed.

On a spring day eleven months earlier, Shannon's world had changed forever. Only moments after dropping her husband, Eric, off at his job, Shannon was broadsided by another car in a terrible accident. When the paramedics arrived, her car was upside down and Shannon was pinned inside. Doctors at the hospital brought bad news to her family and friends assembled outside the intensive care unit: Shannon was alive but paralyzed from the neck down. The force of the collision had damaged her spinal cord and left her a quadriplegic.

Since the accident, Shannon had remained hospitalized. Eric and the rest of her family stayed by her side around the clock, but the stress of Shannon's catastrophic injuries soon began to take its toll on family members. Within weeks of the accident, Eric found himself at odds with Shannon's family, and disagreements arose between Eric and his mother-in-law, Patricia.

Over the next nine months, Shannon continued to deteriorate, but then she rebounded. For several days it looked like she would be well enough to return home as a quadriplegic, until, taking a final turn for the worse, Shannon fell into a coma, lingered for ten weeks, and died. Her doctors determined that her death was the result of systemic bacterial infections, a complication of her accident eleven months earlier.

Because Shannon's death was classified as accidental, related directly to the injuries she sustained in the car accident, Shannon's body was transferred to my morgue, where her case would be reviewed and a death certificate issued. Initially, I did not anticipate the need for an autopsy. She'd been in the hospital for months, and the doctors knew for a long time that her prognosis was poor.

But there was one problem. According to my investigator, Patricia believed her daughter's death had nothing to do with her car accident. Family members said that three months before her death, Shannon became delirious and suddenly refused to take her medications because she was afraid someone was trying to poison her. That "someone," said Patricia, was Eric.

As a forensic pathologist, I know that survivors sometimes experience irrational fears about the causes of their loved ones' deaths. Eric, who was clearly devoted to Shannon, denied the charge. More important, hospital records showed no evidence of foul play. Usually, a simple call from me and an explanation of the medical facts will quell these types of worries, but not always. I tried to explain to Patricia that serious complications often arise from quadriplegia. But she felt strongly that something sinister had happened to her daughter while in the hospital. She blamed Eric.

I decided to comply with Patricia's wishes for an autopsy. I felt we owed it to this woman to try to give her some peace. But providing peace turned out to be a difficult task. I hoped to do it by finding the exact cause of Shannon's sudden turn for the worse and figuring out why she ultimately lapsed into a coma. I did the autopsy not to confirm that she died from the bacterial infections—we knew that—but to see whether there was anything we could point to that would suggest why she became comatose ten weeks earlier. I also hoped the autopsy would uncover a clinical reason behind Shannon's alleged deathbed accusations. The tragic case of Shannon Johnson now became a multilayered mystery.

I started by carefully examining the exterior of Shannon's body, paying close attention to the signs of her long bout with infection. I could plainly see that Shannon suffered from bedsores. Victims of paralysis like Shannon face many life-threatening complications. Most are infections of the lungs or urinary tract, but deadly infections can also be triggered by bedsores. When a person is immobile, the soft tissue covering bones such as the coccyx, spine, hips, and shoulders is compressed by the constant weight of the body, which, if not alleviated, can result in a lack of blood supply to the area. The resulting bedsores can eat away at skin, muscle, and bone, causing bodywide infections. Shannon was also obese, and her obesity exacerbated her bedsores. Increased pressure from her weight caused sores so severe that she developed osteomyelitis, an infection of the bone.

After completing the analysis of the outside of Shannon's body, I began the internal exam. Once the body was opened, fluids were drawn for toxicology tests. But because Shannon's alleged poisoning took place months ago, I would not be able to run screens for poisons. Even though I expected to find evidence of the deadly infections, I was shocked by the extent of the damage; her kidneys and liver had shut down, and her lung cavities were filled with pus.

What killed Shannon was indisputable—systemic bacterial infections, but I still had no answers for Patricia. Why did Shannon claim she was being poisoned, and what could cause her to suddenly fall into a coma?

One organ could perhaps give me the answer: Shannon's brain. After removing Shannon's brain and preserving it in formaldehyde, I turned to Dr. Gary Pearl, a neuropathologist who specializes in diseases of the brain, to see if he could find anything out of the ordinary. During the dissection, Dr. Pearl discovered an abnormality: evidence of damage in her hippocampus, a region of the temporal lobe that plays a role in memory. Moreover, Dr. Pearl was able to estimate that this brain damage occurred approximately two or three months before, about the same time as Shannon's sudden turn for the worse.

Shannon's recurring sequence of infections most likely caused the brain damage. It's not uncommon for blood pressure to drop from serious infections. And that's what I suspect happened. The infection-induced drop in blood pressure diminished blood flow to her brain, causing the brain damage discovered by Dr. Pearl.

Shannon's long descent began on the day of her car accident. During the impact, the force of the collision damaged her spinal cord and left her a quadriplegic. In the hospital, confined to a bed, Shannon developed a series of infections, including severe bedsores. Over the course of nearly a year, her infections grew resistant to almost all antibiotics. She had even lost her hearing due to the toxicity of the powerful antibiotics she'd received. Her infections triggered drops in her blood pressure. During a period of low blood pressure, Shannon's brain was starved of oxygen. Parts of it actually began to die.

Shannon became delusional, possibly because of her episodic low blood pressure, the infections themselves, the medications she was receiving, or even depression. In this state, she accused her husband and others of poisoning her. Then she had a significant hypotensive event that caused her to slip irreversibly into a coma. No longer responsive to antibiotics, infections rapidly spread throughout her body. They destroyed her kidneys and severely damaged her heart, liver, and lungs. Weeks later, Shannon died of the infections, just as the hospital had reported. There was nothing in the hospital records, autopsy, or investigation to suggest that she had been poisoned by her husband or anyone else. I believed I had the most likely explanation for Shannon's clinical course and death. Shannon had died from infections, and there was no poisoning.

Roughly every thirteen minutes, somewhere in the United States, a motor vehicle crash kills. At current mortality rates, a baby born today has roughly one chance in seventy of ultimately dying in a car accident. It is one of those unexpected things that happen, and for the victim's loved ones, each crash is a catastrophic personal tragedy. In my jurisdiction in Florida, where we have some of the deadliest roads in the nation, about one in five of my cases comes from a car crash. Nationally, motor vehicle accidents are the leading cause of death for people of every age from two through thirty-four. As was the case with Shannon

Johnson, fatal accidents have consequences that reverberate through the lives of the victims and their families.

Crash Scene Forensics

For law enforcement, every car accident is a scientific journey, one that begins not in the morgue but out in the field. Florida highway patrolmen investigate more than 3,200 fatal crash scenes per year. Each piece of evidence helps to get at the truth behind an accident.

One of the first things they must do at such a scene is sift through the wreckage. The highway patrol's homicide team is expertly trained to map a scene, taking critical photographs and measurements. They look at skid marks, damage to the vehicles, gouges in the road—anything that might tell the story. The investigators have got to move fast. A rainy night, for example, may wash away portions of a skid mark. At times, the crash site is spread over hundreds of feet. The bodies may no longer be in the car, and it can be difficult to tell who was driving.

Nothing leaves the scene, however, until an investigator from my office gets a firsthand look. All that information arrives with the deceased at the morgue. With every car accident, all the pieces must be put together to come up with what happened. Bad weather, drowsiness, high speed, failing brakes, alcohol, heart attack, seizures, a suicide wish, a murder attempt—every wreck has a story. A car crash may mean the end to a life, but for me, it is just the beginning of an investigation. My discoveries can influence insurance claims, criminal charges, and even future auto designs.

Safer Cars and Roads, but the Same Old Drivers

Nearly forty-three thousand people are killed in motor vehicle accidents annually. Despite this staggering statistic, cars have never been safer than they are today. Between 1980 and 1998, automakers, working to sell more vehicles, engineered a string of safety improvements to protect us from dying in crashes.

When a collision occurs, both the vehicle and the passengers have kinetic energy. As the vehicle decelerates (stops suddenly), the vehicle's kinetic energy and the passengers' kinetic energy must be absorbed. The car's energy is absorbed by mechanical deformation, or crumpling, of its sheet metal. What looks like a mass of tangled metal in a wreck is actually a carefully engineered event, designed to decrease the rate of deceleration during a crash. Engineers want parts of the car to collapse like an accordion in the event of a collision.

Because passengers travel at the same speed as the vehicle, reducing the rate of deceleration also reduces the risk of death and serious injury, even in the most dangerous types of collisions. Seat belts and air bags inside the car manage the remaining deceleration forces, keep the passengers in position, and prevent injuries caused by hitting the steering wheel, windshield, or dashboard. The net effect of these engineering feats has been to reduce crash fatalities by 20 percent.

Other safety innovations include side air bags, antilock brakes, collapsible steering wheels, enhanced exterior lighting, and better restraint devices. Front-impact air bags now include sensors that identify children and smaller adults. The air bag deploys with less force to minimize injuries to those passengers. Even seemingly small changes can make a difference: Equipping cars with center rear brake lights, for example, has actually decreased rear-end collisions by 4 percent.

Sound amazing? You ain't seen nothing yet! A super-high-tech age of auto safety is dawning in which cars will protect us like tanks in even the most violent crashes. Coming soon is even more advanced "crash avoidance" technology, with devices like electronic sensors that will detect danger ahead and then steer you out of harm's way; systems to help you control the distance between your car and the vehicle in front of you; and cameras to give you a better view as you back into tight parking spots and perform other visibility-limited maneuvers. Safer tires are on the way, too, designed to run flat-free for longer distances. Such safety innovations won't come cheap; many are already available in luxury cars.

Over time, however, automakers promise this technology will become standard over a broader, more affordable range of cars.

Our roads are also safer these days, with better use of reflector lights, well-spaced traffic signals, widely separated lanes, gentler curves, improved signs, and less-slippery road surfaces. Combating death on America's highways has certainly been a technological and engineering success.

Yet, despite these wonderful innovations, traffic fatalities continue to rise. Why? In the end, it's not so much the car you drive as how you drive it. Human error remains the chief cause of car accidents. You can't engineer for bad decisions and bad driving habits.

How Not to Die in a Car Crash

Most people have never seen what a fatal car crash can do to a body, but I see it almost every day. The injuries from car accidents can be absolutely brutal: Deceleration forces can be so intense that your insides will try to pass through your outsides. I've seen bodies with aortas sliced apart, diaphragms ripped in half, abdominal organs that have landed in the chest cavity, and head injuries in which the top of the head is torn from the first cervical vertebrae. Some injuries are so overwhelming that they look like a bad horror flick, and to the uninitiated, they can be a real stomach churner.

Could faster, better trauma care help reduce such horrific deaths, or could the reduction come about mostly through injury prevention, or both?

Several years ago, I collaborated on a study with a group of trauma surgeons at the University of Texas Health Science Center to help answer these questions. We classified 753 highway deaths as "therapeutically not preventable," "possibly preventable," or "preventable." We also reviewed the accident victims' charts, searching for factors such as intoxication, seat belt use, and motorcycle helmet use that might have prevented or lessened the severity of their injuries. The primary causes of death included brain and spinal cord injuries; irreversible shock;

multiple injuries; multiple organ failure or infection; and in a few cases, pulmonary embolism (clots in the lungs).

Our study concluded that only 13 percent of fatal accident victims could have possibly survived with improved trauma care, such as preventing multiorgan failure, stemming infection, or preventing clots. The remaining victims had unsalvageable injuries. Here's the deal: Although wonderful advancements have been made in trauma care, injury prevention remains the only way to reduce deaths on our highways.

In fact, most highway deaths are so preventable that traffic experts don't even refer to them as "accidents" anymore. They use the term "collisions." Ask any police officer or traffic investigator and you will find that nearly every collision they have ever worked was in some way avoidable. You don't have to be in (or die from) an automobile accident if you drive defensively at all times. Nor do you have to put others at risk. Here's how.

Decelerate from Death

I see far too many collisions caused by excessive speed. With every ten miles per hour faster you go, your risk of dying goes up proportionately. So don't speed! You don't save that much time. Slowing down means my son will be ten minutes late for band practice instead of eight—but I won't risk injuring or killing anyone. The choice is obvious.

Resist the urge to accelerate on yellow (amber) lights. Most traffic signals are only thirty to fifty seconds long. Rushing through an intersection can put your life at risk.

Never speed through parking lots, either. They have pedestrians.

Please Fasten Your Seats Belts

There are people who would be alive today had they worn their seat belts. (In the crash that killed Princess Diana the only survivor was the one wearing a seat belt.)

If I can double my chances of surviving an accident by buckling up, why not?

Seat belts work because they keep drivers and passengers in their vehicles.

If you're in a vehicle crash, there's a lot of structure around you. The interior of your car is a far more forgiving environment than the outside of your car. When you're ejected from a vehicle in a crash, bad things happen.

Just as important, you've got to use restraints the way they were engineered. If you wear a lap belt without the shoulder harness, for example, you're in danger of life-threatening internal injuries. I've seen people who were almost cut in half by the lap belt because they didn't use the shoulder harness. The harness helps keep the body and organs in sync and off the dashboard. If a seat back is reclined, the restraint becomes much less effective, if not useless, because the shoulder harness moves away from the passenger.

Air bags save lives, too. Safety experts recommend that seats should be moved back as far as possible for air bags to offer the best protection and cushioning when they deploy.

Keep Your Kids Safe

- For the best possible protection, keep your infant in the back seat, in a rear-facing child safety seat, as long as possible up to the height or weight limit of the particular seat—usually until a minimum of age one and at least twenty pounds.

- When infants outgrow their rear-facing seats, they should ride in the back seat in forward-facing child safety seats, until they reach the upper weight or height limit of the particular seat (usually around age four and forty pounds).

- Once your kids outgrow their forward-facing seats, they should ride in booster seats, in the back seat, until the vehicle seat belts fit properly. Seat belts fit properly when the lap belt lays across the upper thighs and the shoulder belt fits across the chest.

- When your kids outgrow their booster seats, (usually at age eight or when they are four feet nine inches tall), they can use the adult seat belt in the back seat, if it fits properly.

Source: National Highway Traffic Safety Administration

Pulling Over: A Deadly Driving Mistake

Often, car accident victims are simply in the wrong place at the wrong time. I never, ever stop my car on the side of a freeway, for example. I've had cases in which drivers did this to fix a flat tire and were rear-ended and killed. I've had two cases in which police officers were killed that way.

If something goes wrong with your car, don't pull over until you can get to an off-ramp, side street, or gas station. Once, when I was on the freeway, my engine light came on. My son wanted me to stop the car. I knew that an illuminated engine light wasn't going to kill me, but that stopping on the side of the freeway might, so I waited until I could drive to a safer location to check it out.

Driving While Distracted

For some people, a car is the perfect place to apply makeup, talk on the phone, and guzzle coffee—while trying to keep an eye on the road and a hand on the wheel. These days, some people also think it's a good spot to send text messages. But anything that distracts you from driving can have terrible consequences. Driver inattentiveness causes about 25 percent of all car crashes in the United States. Once I autopsied a young, beautiful girl who had died in a car crash. Witnesses said she took her eyes off the road to fiddle with her CD player. In that split second, she lost control of her car and smashed into a steel barrier.

Other attention stealers include rubbernecking (particularly looking at roadside accidents!), getting distracted by passengers (think small kids), and using cell phones. By the way, it's not so much the yakking on a cell phone as it is the content of the conversation. An argument with your spouse, for example, is more likely to interfere with your focus and reaction time than, say, a quick call to say that you got off work late.

I know what inattentiveness will do. One of the few times I've ever been in an accident was when I was pulling out of my garage while yelling at my son. I crashed straight into my husband's car in the driveway.

Sometimes distractions are unavoidable. I had one poor fellow—a truck driver—who died when a bee flew into his cab, which is why I recommend driving with the windows rolled up. And if not rolled up, then roll them all the way down. Windows rolled halfway down can cause the most traumatic injuries if you get partially thrown from your car.

Keep your eyes on the road and concentrate on your driving. This includes looking down the road and anticipating what is ahead. Scan your side and rearview mirrors every several seconds. Know your blind spots and adjust for them. When it can be done safely, look not only at cars around you but at their drivers as well. Information such as the age of a driver and their attentiveness— whether they are talking on the phone, shaving, or so forth—can alert you to potential hazards.

> **TURN THE TABLES:** Beware of Flying Objects
>
> Anything unrestrained in your car can become a dangerous missile: groceries, jumper cables, sports equipment, and plenty of other items. Put them into trunk organizers designed especially for your car.

Don't Let Friends (or Yourself) Drive Drunk

It sounds like a cliché, but there's a strong, indisputable link between blood alcohol concentration and the risk of a crash. With his red hair and freckles, nineteen-year-old Jimmy Fredericks looked like the all-American kid who would never get into any trouble. When he was arrested for drunk driving, his parents were shocked. But somehow, he beat the DUI charge. On the last night of his life, he decided to celebrate his legal victory. He stopped at a convenience store and persuaded someone to buy him a six-pack of beer. Doing about sixty miles per hour on the suburban streets of Orlando, he lost control and slammed into a tree so hard that his car snapped in two. He was killed instantly. I met him the next morning—at the morgue.

Alcohol impairs driving capability, and the more serious the crash, the more likely that alcohol was involved. At least 40 percent of people who die in traffic accidents have alcohol in their systems. I wouldn't go anywhere near the wheel of a car after having even a glass of wine, because one glass does me in.

LIFE LESSONS: The 8 Leading Driver Mistakes That Cause Collisions

1. Excessive speed
2. Right-of-way violations
3. Improper turning
4. Improper passing
5. Following too closely (tailgating)
6. Driving left of center
7. Alcohol/substance abuse
8. Distracted drivers

Source: National Highway Traffic Safety Administration

Dead-on-Your-Feet Driving

Drowsy drivers account for about one hundred thousand accidents a year. These are usually single-vehicle accidents, though some are terrible head-on collisions.

Another of my cases, student Jeremy Decker, age twenty-one, was driving back to Florida State in Tallahassee, after attending a wedding in Miami. He wanted to get back to classes and decided to drive through the night. After stopping at a fast-food restaurant for a high-carbohydrate breakfast, Jeremy got back on the highway. Shortly thereafter, his car left the roadway, struck an embankment, and burst into flames. He died in the inferno. He had no alcohol in his system, and, as best as we could tell, there was nothing mechanically wrong with his car. We concluded that he had fallen asleep at the wheel.

Before taking a road trip, be sure to get a good night's sleep. On a long trip, it's a good idea to have at least two drivers who can take turns. If you're driving, don't ignore signs of sleepiness such as yawning, a sensation of heavy eyelids, difficulty focusing your eyes, trouble keeping your head up, and so forth. Pull into a rest stop and take a nap. On long trips, take frequent breaks, at least once every two hours or every one hundred miles. Having a big meal or one loaded with carbohydrates will make you drowsy, so avoid those and opt for light, protein-rich snacks instead. Drinking a cup of coffee or two helps, too. Even though I'm a terrible singer—I've been asked by my family not to belt out tunes in the shower—I've found it helpful on solo drives to play CDs and sing along with them to stay alert.

Bad Drive Times

The most dangerous hours to be on the roadways are Friday night and Saturday night between midnight and 3 a.m. (when the bars typically close). Personally, I'm not a late-night gal anyway, but I make sure to stay off the road then. One of my sons hasn't started driving yet, but after he gets his license, he's not going to be happy when I make him avoid those times, too.

LIFE LESSONS: Motorists and Pedestrians Face Greater Risks Than Airline Travelers

What fascinates me is not that the world is so full of risks, but that we're so bad at assessing them. Most of the things we fear, like crashing in an airplane, are unlikely to ever happen to us. In fact, the chances of dying in an airplane crash are just 1 in 5,552. Statistically, you are much more likely to be killed in a car crash, where the chance of death is 1 in 84. Also, your lifetime risk of being killed by a motor vehicle if you're a pedestrian is 1 in 631. Your chance of dying after being hit by a car going 20 mph is 5 percent; 30 mph, 40 percent; 40 mph, 80 percent; and at 50 mph or faster, 100 percent.

Are You an Emotional Driver?

You're at much greater risk of injuries or death if you join in a traffic dispute, even if it's by honking your horn or glaring at another driver—habits that many men, in particular, find hard to resist. Anyone who raises a middle finger is playing Russian roulette on the road.

Drivers who are antagonistic and stressed are ready to fight when they get behind the wheel. Their reactions to other drivers who argue or act angry toward them can result in fatal crashes, if not other violent outcomes. Aggressive drivers, who are overwhelmingly more likely to be males, attack others with perhaps the most dangerous weapon of all—their own cars.

I've seen what happens when traffic disputes turn deadly. On a stretch of Orlando highway in summer 2007, Ray Strickland was driving to work on his morning commute when he got into a driving duel. Another driver, Hank MacLaren, had cut him off, and they exited the highway onto a city street. Hank pulled up next to Ray at a red light, got out of his car, started cursing, then began pounding on Ray's window. Ray got out of his car, and Hank shot and killed him. My advice: Never underestimate another driver's ability to commit mayhem—or murder.

Intersection Smarts

More than 65 percent of all traffic collisions occur at or are influenced by an intersection, says the National Highway Traffic Safety Administration (NHTSA). The average speed of a driver passing through an intersection is over 50 mph! That makes intersections very dangerous places to be. Yet, we often carelessly race through them. Crashes at intersections are among the most fatal, because they tend to be T-bone (broadside) crashes in which seat belts and air bags are less effective. On the other hand, you can eliminate nearly seven out of ten chances of being involved in a collision merely by being particularly alert at intersections!

Also, never enter an intersection without being able to pass through it unimpeded. It's extremely hazardous to enter one, then have to stop and yield to oncoming traffic. This is a common occurrence when vehicles make left turns at intersections. Once a decision is reached to initiate a left-hand turn, attempt to complete the turn as quickly and as safely as possible, minimizing your exposure to an intersection's lines of traffic.

Traffic Sense

Protect yourself in traffic. Travel in the center or right lane and allow plenty of room on all four sides of your vehicle. If other vehicles crowd you or tailgate, adjust for their poor driving skills. That way, you give yourself options in the event of an emergency. It's easier to avoid poor drivers when they are in front of you. Allow them to pass. Always use your turn signals, too. Let other drivers know what your intentions are. Don't assume the same courtesy from them.

Know When to Turn Over Your Keys

Per mile, drivers over the age of seventy-five have more accidents than any other group except teenagers. Florida, where I live and work, is most affected by this. We have the largest population of elderly people in the nation—18 percent—and, not surprisingly, the highest number of auto fatalities. In an effort to reduce elderly death rates, Florida passed a law in 2006 requiring vision tests for drivers ages seventy-nine and older when renewing licenses.

Although driving skills tend to start slipping at about age sixty-five, most older drivers recognize that fact and make adjustments to their driving styles. They may give up night driving, skip rush-hour traffic, or go around the block to avoid left-hand turns at intersections (something I've been doing since I was sixteen years old), which are the leading site of accidents. The challenge is to identify older people who drive poorly and don't compensate for their faults, and drive defensively around them.

Road Kill

Age and driving skill were factors in a case involving eighty-one-year-old Ricardo Sanchez, found dead in his apartment one morning. According to the known facts, friends and family last saw Ricardo four days earlier when he left a small get-together just before dusk. He didn't like driving at night because of his age, and he had some minor eye problems.

We learned from his family that Ricardo was an energetic man with a great sense of humor. During the last several years of his life, he spent much of his time with his close-knit family enjoying his retirement. Like many in retirement, Ricardo, who had lived alone since his divorce ten years earlier, clung to his independence. He insisted on driving rather than relying upon others for transportation. He also refused any professional home care, despite having severe coronary artery disease, high blood pressure, and diabetes. As far as his family and friends knew, Ricardo made it home safely that evening. Four days later, however, no one had heard from him. Ricardo's son and sister found him face-down on the floor, wearing the same outfit he had on at the family get-together.

At first, Ricardo's death was classified as natural and his body was transferred to a funeral home for burial, but hours later his family made a startling discovery, one that raised new suspicions. His car was missing.

Was he a victim of foul play? I decided to retrieve his body from the funeral home, do some X-rays, and examine him externally for any signs of trauma. I didn't find anything out of the ordinary, so I didn't perform a full autopsy. We returned Ricardo's body to the funeral home.

The vast majority of the deaths that fall into the jurisdiction of the District Nine morgue don't require autopsies. We get thousands of calls about elderly people who have died. I don't need to autopsy most of them because it's cost prohibitive for the county. Forensic autopsies are done only in certain circumstances, including cases involving criminal violence, homicide, suicide, accidents, or suspicious or unusual circumstances. The latter would include the death of someone without a significant medical history, or when someone dies in jail or while in police custody. An autopsy would not be done, therefore, if you died from medical causes, such as heart disease, emphysema, or cancer, and there was medical history to support the diagnosis—unless there was something suspicious about the death.

Just hours after Ricardo's body was released from the morgue, the Orlando Police Department called me with surprising information. Ricardo's vehicle had been located in an auto wrecker lot. The elderly man was apparently not a victim of foul play but involved in a car accident the day of his death. Given the unusual circumstances surrounding Ricardo's death and to bring closure to his family, I decided to perform a full autopsy. The body was immediately transported from a local funeral home to the morgue—for a second time.

From the autopsy and other facts, I figured out what had happened to Ricardo Sanchez and why he had died. After leaving his family and friends, he drove home sometime near dusk. Only a few miles from his home, Ricardo's trip was cut short. Apparently, he tried to make a left-hand turn and was hit by an oncoming car.

The force of the impact caused a subdural hematoma, bleeding in the brain that occurs under the dura mater, the protective membrane that covers the brain. With that single finding, I could see with certainty what killed Ricardo Sanchez—a significant head injury. And I also knew how the fatal trauma occurred: the car accident.

Had he requested medical attention at the scene, Ricardo might have survived, but he likely did not realize the severity of his condition—for two reasons. Initially, the bleeding can be slow and not cause any problems. Also, like many elderly individuals, Ricardo's brain had shrunken with age and was actually better able to accommodate the bleeding.

One of the messiest challenges for adult children and their parents to navigate is the driving question. When an elderly parent's driving gets dangerously erratic, a serious talk about hanging up the keys becomes necessary. Be persistent if you're the adult child, and realistic if you're the parent. The concern is about safety—yours and that of others.

Whenever I see victims of a motor vehicle crash, I think, "They should not be dead." I see the tragic results of these crashes every day, and of course it has impacted me. I'm always on my kids' cases about safety: Watch out for careless drivers, don't speed, never get in a car with an irresponsible driver or someone who's been drinking—all that. My work prompts me to resolve to become a better driver every time I get behind the wheel. And it reminds me, once again, that life is the most precious thing we have.

Stay Alive: Motorcycle Safety Tips

For motorcyclists, the dangers are greater than for motorists. A motorcyclist is thirty-seven times more likely to die in a motor vehicle crash than someone in a car. Here are a few safety tips:

- Wear a good helmet. An unhelmeted rider is much more likely to suffer severe or fatal head trauma in a crash than a helmeted rider. Many motorcyclists want a choice, though. Let me suggest one: When you ride, strap on either a helmet or a dunce cap.
- Wear riding attire that's designed to protect against abrasion and impact.
- Avoid heavy traffic. Stay off busy highways and instead take back roads that are less crowded.
- Assume you are invisible to all other drivers on the road at all times, and ride defensively.
- Never pull knot-headed stunts, like weaving in and out of traffic.
- If you're an inexperienced rider, or haven't been on a motorcycle in a long time, take a motorcycle safety refresher course and get some practice in a deserted parking lot. Additionally, get to know the handling characteristics of your bike.

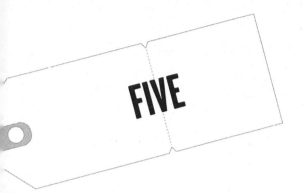

FIVE

Dead Weight

Heavy Risks

The body lying before me came in from a local emergency room, wrapped in white hospital sheets. She was young, just twenty-eight years old, and the resident of a homeless shelter in Orlando. Of all the bodies that come to my morgue every year, one out of fifteen is homeless. Seldom do they have a medical history to help me figure out how they died.

This one was an exception, however, and came with medical records. Hers weren't particularly revealing, but I burrowed into them anyway. She had a history of high blood pressure and was supposedly eleven weeks pregnant. She did not smoke or use drugs. Puzzling to me was that she had told the shelter staff that she was suffering from ovarian cancer. I couldn't get that information substantiated in her medical records.

Working in forensics obliges me to describe a person's racial origin, primarily for identification purposes. This woman was Caucasian, and her name was Veronica Murphy. Really, I knew little more about her except that she was dead—and very heavy, 340 pounds, which is considered morbidly obese. A person is characterized as morbidly obese if they weigh more than double their ideal body weight, or are 100 pounds or more overweight.

Approximately three hundred thousand Americans will die prematurely from obesity this year, and millions more will know its agony. Anyone who puts on pounds year after year is at risk for becoming overweight, obese, or even morbidly obese, unless this gradual process of weight gain is nipped in the bud. It's a short road from being overweight (like most Americans are) to becoming officially obese.

Nearly 25 percent of American kids are either overweight or obese. Some scientists believe that today's generation of overweight children will have shorter life spans than their parents. Things haven't been moving in such a positive direction globally, either. It's estimated that 250 million people worldwide are obese. If current trends continue, the battle of the bulge will overtake smoking as the primary cause of preventable death.

But whether Veronica Murphy's weight had anything to do with her death was unclear. When a case comes to my morgue in which the deceased is overweight or obese, a long list of possibilities exists as to why he or she died.

This was a sad case, to be sure. My investigator reported that Veronica had arrived at the homeless shelter with her six-year-old son and six-month-old infant in tow, after fleeing an abusive relationship and falling on hard times. She was filled with hope and ready to put her struggles behind her. Six days after checking in to the shelter, though, Veronica suddenly fell to the floor, unconscious. Paramedics arrived. As she was wheeled into the ambulance, she opened her eyes and told her young son, "Mommy will be okay. Mommy will be right back."

She couldn't have been more wrong. Before arriving at the emergency room, Veronica was dead.

My fact-finding mission into her death began with an external examination of her body. I wanted to determine first whether there were any signs of trauma, since she had reportedly been a victim of domestic violence. There were none. After taking measurements and weighing the body, we took photographs from every angle.

The next major part of the autopsy was the internal examination. There was no evidence of cancer in her ovaries, only some cysts, but these were benign and wouldn't have caused her death.

With ovarian cancer ruled out as a cause of death, I wanted to see if she was pregnant when she died. I carefully examined her womb without breaking open the amniotic sac. Inside I could see a fetus. It looked normally developed and was about two inches long. From that I could fairly estimate that Veronica was about eleven to twelve weeks pregnant. She had become pregnant only three months after giving birth to her second child.

These facts raised a red flag. Overweight and obese women are more than twice as likely as normal-weight women to suffer a dangerous blood clot in the lungs during pregnancy. Many times you don't even know you're in danger until it's too late.

But the minute I saw Veronica's heart, I wondered if she had died of something other than a blood clot. A normal heart is about as big as a fist. Hers was double that size—the biggest heart I'd seen in a long time. An enlarged heart is often attributed to high blood pressure, known medically as hypertension. With high blood pressure, the heart must work harder to push blood through the arteries. This never-ending workout causes the heart to grow. But unlike other muscles in the body, bigger isn't necessarily better. An enlarged heart can place undue strain on the muscle and result in sudden cardiac arrest.

Size wasn't the only problem with Veronica's heart. It also contained patches of scar tissue, medically known as fibrosis. Portions of her heart tissue had previously been destroyed and replaced by scarring. This was uncommon in someone so young.

The whole case could have ended right there, except for one thing. I found enormous blood clots in her lungs. They were elongated, roughly the size of fingers and dark red in color. Finally, I had all the pieces of the puzzle. I began putting them together to reconstruct Veronica's final moments.

When she checked in to the shelter, Veronica had two serious risk factors for developing deadly blood clots: morbid obesity and an eleven-week pregnancy.

Her circulation needed help to get the venous blood back up to her heart. Under normal circumstances, assistance comes from the muscles in the legs. They help pump blood toward the heart by squeezing the deep veins in the legs. But when you're obese, you don't have enough muscle to do this, so blood pools in the veins, and clots may form. When a dangerous blood clot forms deep in the leg muscles, it is called a deep vein thrombosis. The clot sometimes breaks free and floats into the lungs, and may cause sudden death. A deep vein clot is not to be confused with blood clots that form on atherosclerotic plaque in arteries and block the flow of blood to the brain, causing a stroke; or to the heart, causing a heart attack.

In Veronica's case, several large, deep leg clots broke free. They were swiftly pumped up into the heart and straight into the pulmonary artery, which supplies blood to the lungs for oxygenation. A clot lodged there and shut off the flow of blood to the lungs, leading to cardiac arrest. Veronica was killed by a pulmonary embolism. Even though her unhealthy heart and high blood pressure could have killed her at any time with a deadly arrhythmia (an irregular heartbeat), the blood clots trumped that. Large pulmonary emboli that block the blood flow to both lungs are incompatible with life.

Could Veronica's premature death have been prevented? Possibly, had she been under a doctor's care. Doctors can identify risk factors like obesity that can slow down blood flow and set the stage for clot formation. They can also diagnose blood clots through sophisticated tests such as sonograms, treat them with anticoagulants, and reduce further risk of clot formation.

After ruling on Veronica's death, I called her family, as I do with many of my cases. This was one of those situations where the family had no opportunity to say good-bye, and my heart went out to them. The best I could do was make sure they understood what had happened. Hopefully, my words would help them come to grips with their sudden, tragic loss. Her young children, thankfully, found a safe, loving home with Veronica's relatives.

Obesity wouldn't be such a big deal if the problem were just cosmetic, but it's not. Excessive weight takes a terrible toll on the body and can shave up to twenty years off your life. Whenever I open up a body that is heavy, I am witness to the damage obesity does. I see the visible effects of high blood pressure in what is called left ventricular hypertrophy, or thickening of the left side of the heart. I see the yellow-tinged granules of cholesterol that collect in coronary arteries as plaque. I see the sacs of diverticulosis in the colons of those who eat little fiber and rarely exercise. And in cases like Veronica's, I run across deadly clots.

It's very difficult for people who are obese to be completely healthy. They run a significantly higher risk of coronary heart disease, stroke, high blood pressure, some cancers, diabetes, gout, arthritis, gallstones, infertility, injuries due to falls and lifting, and childbirth complications than do people of normal weight. But that's not all. There are not-so-familiar diseases like sleep apnea and fatty liver disease, both potentially deadly. Sleep apnea occurs when you stop breathing momentarily many times throughout the night because your airways become blocked when muscles in your throat relax. Anatomical problems such as fat around the pharynx contribute to the problem. Obesity is a risk factor for sleep apnea, and 30 percent of people with a BMI over 30 will have obstructive sleep apnea. Left untreated, sleep apnea can increase the risk of heart attack, stroke, and high blood pressure. Many times you don't know you have it unless your bedmate notices it or hears you snoring loudly. Weight loss is one of the simpler treatments for sleep apnea.

More and more obese people are turning up with fatty liver disease, a buildup of fat in the liver cells that usually causes no damage. However, there's a more serious type called nonalcoholic steatohepatitis, or NASH, that causes liver inflammation and, sometimes, the formation of fibrous (scar) tissue. In some cases, this can lead to either cirrhosis, which is progressive, irreversible liver scarring, or liver cancer.

The connection between obesity and some of these conditions and illnesses has not been proven scientifically beyond a shadow of a doubt. But we do know this: When you lose weight—even as little as 10 to 15 percent of your weight—these problems get better. This suggests that obesity plays a big role in their development.

I'm not trying to frighten anyone, but I want you to be aware of something else: For someone hugely overweight, minor surgery becomes major surgery and infinitely more risky. Some of these increased risks include difficulty with intubation and anesthesia, poor wound healing, increased risk of infection, and post-surgical blood clots, not to mention the technical difficulties the surgeon often encounters due to the fatty tissue itself. I recall a case in which an overweight middle-aged woman had undergone knee replacement surgery (obesity causes wear and tear on your joints), only to drop dead a few days later. Her death was a riddle to me until I unmasked an unusual killer: Fat globules from her bone marrow traveled to her lungs and caused sudden death. Though her fat embolism was not directly related to her obesity, the reason for her surgery was. There's no such thing as risk-free surgery, but it's even more risky if you're heavy.

Then there's the day-to-day misery of just trying to live life. Imagine how hard it is for a wide body to squeeze into a narrow armchair, strap on undersized seat belts, or go through a turnstile. It's much more difficult to maintain personal hygiene if you're obese. Believe it or not, I've found items like remote controls and packages of cigarettes in people's fat rolls.

I've seen a trend toward fatter bodies in my morgue, which creates logistical problems for me as a medical examiner. Years ago, I autopsied a nine-hundred-pound woman and had to place her body on two side-by-side autopsy tables to get the job done. Today, we use bigger (and more expensive) autopsy tables, with hydraulic pumps to help us lift these very heavy bodies. Once I start an autopsy on an obese person, it makes for a difficult, messy procedure. So much fat tissue is in the body (think big globules that look like mounds of yellow tapioca pudding), that it's a startling sight to someone seeing it for the first time, and it's like working in a vat of grease. Scalpels can slide out of your hands, and that's dangerous. Funeral directors have told me that people who are very obese when they die often cannot be cremated because the body won't fit in the cremation chamber or the volume of fat could ignite a fire that could spread beyond the chamber. The obesity problem has definitely spilled over into the morgue and death industry. But that's not what's most important here: You are.

Weighty Matters

The pressing issue is that obesity is a health risk and cuts lives short. But what constitutes risk? Your body mass index, or BMI, is a number doctors use to determine whether you're at a healthy weight. It's basically a ratio of weight to height. Anything between 18.5 and 24.9 is considered healthy. Anything above 25 is overweight and potentially unhealthy; above 30 is definitely obese and puts you at increased risk of dying prematurely. The chart on page 108 shows you how to figure BMI, or use an online calculator, such as the one at www.cdc.gov. It quickly figures your BMI after you plug in your measurements.

Adult BMI Chart and Other Ways to Measure Obesity

One problem with BMI is that it does a poor job of taking body type and muscle mass into consideration, meaning that a tall, muscular person can be labeled obese. A good example is David Robinson, formerly of the San Antonio Spurs basketball team. Our sons went to the same school, so I'd often see him. Robinson had a well-chiseled physique, but at seven feet one inch tall and 250 pounds, his BMI would be around 25, making him one of the "fattest" players in the NBA. But not really. BMI is an imperfect measure, but it can give you a fairly accurate picture of where you stand, if you're not an athlete.

Many doctors use additional methods to evaluate risk. Waist circumference, for example, is a good way to detect dangerous visceral fat—the kind that pads internal organs and creates potbellies, inviting heart disease, stroke, and diabetes (and making autopsies hard to do). Men with waists over forty inches and women with waists over thirty-five inches are the likeliest to have problems. Fat on your hips and buttocks isn't quite as dangerous as fat around the abdomen, although it can increase your risk of degenerative arthritis, a disabling joint disease that affects millions of people. There are other ways to check your weight: Step on the scale, look at yourself in the mirror, or feel how your clothes fit. I think we know when we're getting fat.

Locate your height in the left-hand column. Read across the row to match that height with your weight. Follow that column up to the top row to find your BMI.

BMI	19	20	21	22	23	24	25	26	27	28	29	30	31	32	33	34	35
Height							Weight in Pounds										
4'10"	91	96	100	105	110	115	119	124	129	134	138	143	148	153	158	162	167
4'11"	94	99	104	109	114	119	124	128	133	138	143	148	153	158	163	168	173
5'	97	102	107	112	118	123	128	133	138	143	148	153	158	163	168	174	179
5'1"	100	106	111	116	122	127	132	137	143	148	153	158	164	169	174	180	185
5'2"	104	109	115	120	126	131	136	142	147	153	158	164	169	175	180	186	191
5'3"	107	113	118	124	130	135	141	146	152	158	163	169	175	180	186	191	197
5'4"	110	116	122	128	134	140	145	151	157	163	169	174	180	186	192	197	204
5'5"	114	120	126	132	138	144	150	156	162	168	174	180	186	192	198	204	210
5'6"	118	124	130	136	142	148	155	161	167	173	179	186	192	198	204	210	216
5'7"	121	127	134	140	146	153	159	166	172	178	185	191	198	204	211	217	223
5'8"	125	131	138	144	151	158	164	171	177	184	190	197	203	210	216	223	230
5'9"	128	135	142	149	155	162	169	176	182	189	196	203	209	216	223	230	236
5'10"	132	139	146	153	160	167	174	181	188	195	202	209	216	222	229	236	243
5'11"	136	143	150	157	165	172	179	186	193	200	208	215	222	229	236	243	250
6'	140	147	154	162	169	177	184	191	199	206	213	221	228	235	242	250	258
6'1"	144	151	159	166	174	182	189	197	204	212	219	227	235	242	250	257	265
6'2"	148	155	163	171	179	186	194	202	210	218	225	233	241	249	256	264	272
6'3"	152	160	168	176	184	192	200	208	216	224	232	240	248	256	264	272	279
	Healthy Weight						Overweight					Obese					

Source: Evidence Report of Clinical Guidelines on the Identification, Evaluation, and Treatment of Overweight and Obesity in Adults, 1998. NIH/National Heart, Lung, and Blood Institute (NHLBI).

Why We're Fat

So why is obesity happening? The obvious, clichéd-but-true answer is that we eat too much high-calorie food and don't burn it off with enough exercise. If only we had more willpower, the problem would go away. But it isn't that easy.

When warned about the dangers of overeating, we get briefly spooked and try to do better. Then we're offered a plateful of pancakes smothered in maple syrup, our appetite overpowers our reason, and before we know it, we're at it again. Just why is appetite such a powerful driver of behavior, and, more important, how can we tame it?

Within the past few years, science has linked our ravenous appetites to genes and hormones. Among the hormones that fuel these urges are ghrelin and leptin, known as the "hunger hormones." Ghrelin is produced mostly by cells in the stomach lining. Its job is to make you feel hungry by affecting the hypothalamus, which governs metabolism. Ghrelin levels rise in dieters who lose weight and then try to keep it off. It's almost as if their bodies are trying to regain the lost fat. This is one reason why it's hard to lose weight and maintain the loss.

Leptin turns your appetite off and is made by fat cells. Low leptin levels increase your appetite and signal your body to store more fat. High leptin levels relay the opposite signal. Many obese people have developed a resistance to the appetite-suppressing effects of leptin and never feel satisfied, no matter how much they eat. Basically, your body uses these hormones to help you stay at your weight and keep you from losing fat—which is another reason why dieting can be so difficult.

Lack of sleep promotes obesity by messing with these hunger hormones. If you skimp on sleep, ghrelin levels rise, making you hungry, and leptin levels dip, which signals a need for calories. During my internship, I was chronically sleep-deprived because I had to be at the hospital and stay up all night every third night. I gained a lot of weight that year; now I know why. Years later, after I gave birth to my son Alex, I put on a lot of pounds, too—twenty pounds left over from the pregnancy, and twenty pounds from being up all night with him. He had colic (fussiness) and never slept more than twenty minutes at a time the first six months of his life. My weight started coming off more easily when I got more sleep.

Besides ghrelin and leptin, many other hormones play a role in appetite. Scientists have been looking for ways to control all these hunger hormones, but so far nothing usable has panned out.

Hunger isn't the only reason people eat and eat and eat. Stress, depression, boredom, loneliness, and even joy all come into play. And some of us may just be inclined to gain weight while others are not, due to genetics. Scientists are unclear as to how much of a role genetics plays in how chubby you are, but estimates range from as low as 20 percent to as high as 90 percent. In studies of twins, researchers have found that siblings wind up with similar body weights, whether or not they are raised in different families, and that adopted children are much more likely to grow to the size of their natural parents than their adoptive ones. Scientists speculate that part of the reason so many of us are susceptible to layering on fat is due to the "thrifty gene." Supposedly, it's a gene passed down from our prehistoric ancestors who could eat a lot and build up reserves of fat to survive frequent famines. Genetically, this made sense when you didn't know if your next meal would be tomorrow or a week from now, but when your next meal is whenever you drive by a fast-food restaurant, that's a problem.

Another cause of obesity, one that really fascinates me, has to do with a virus called the adenovirus-36. It comes from the family of common viruses that causes colds, pneumonia, diarrhea, and pinkeye and is present in 30 percent of obese people and 5 percent of non-obese people. Scientists found that when human stem cells are exposed to adenovirus-36, they turn into fat cells. This discovery is more evidence that our expanding waistlines are due to factors other than weak willpower and, theoretically, could lead to the development of a vaccine to prevent obesity.

Often, hard-to-budge weight is a symptom of a hidden medical problem. You could have hypothyroidism (sluggish thyroid function), a condition that slows down your metabolism and makes it tough to lose weight, or Cushing's disease, characterized by high levels of the hormone cortisol in the blood. A glut of cortisol triggers weight gain, mostly in the trunk and face. Some women have polycystic ovary syndrome (PCOS), a treatable condition that involves a hormone imbalance. And about 30 percent of people who are obese have binge-eating disorders. Sufferers don't just munch on a few potato chips, they inhale the whole bag, and they do this kind of thing habitually. Even certain medications, some of which may be sitting in your medicine cabinet right now, can put on pounds. Common offenders include some antidepressants like Paxil and Zoloft; mood stabilizers; diabetes drugs; blood pressure agents; steroids; anti-seizure drugs; certain hormones; and antihistamines.

So perhaps there is a medical issue that spells weight trouble, or our genes and hormones may be conspiring to makes us eat more, or maybe we're infected with a virus that makes us fat. Should we throw up our hands and say, "Well, I can't do anything about it, so I'll just stay fat"? No, because obesity will affect your health, and it may kill you eventually. You will just have to work a little harder to get your weight under control.

> **LIFE LESSONS**: Fat Cells Are Active, Not Passive
>
> We tend to think of lowly fat cells—those building blocks of flab—as passive, inert entities, but they are, in fact, active and smarter than anyone ever suspected. Fat tissue is an endocrine organ that secretes hormones and other substances (including leptin) with profound and sometimes harmful effects on metabolism, weight, and overall health—another reason for keeping your weight under control.

How Not to Die from Overweight or Obesity

Clearly, obesity is complicated—a condition caused by genes, hormones, environment, physiology, and psychology—and not necessarily by poor willpower or a lack of trying. I find it reassuring to know this because it helps me have more resolve when dealing with my own frustrating ups and downs in weight. Obesity doesn't respond to a quick fix, or a one-size-fits all program. It has multiple causes, so you have to tackle it with multiple strategies. Here's how:

See Your Doc

Obesity is a medical problem that may require a medical solution. If you're adding on extra pounds and don't know why, or if you're having trouble losing weight, see a doctor you trust—preferably someone board certified in internal medicine or family practice. Your doctor can track down the problem and rule out disease-induced weight gain by running various lab tests and conducting a physical exam. Remember, too, that there are complications related to obesity—from heart disease to elevated blood sugar to sleep apnea—and these must be addressed and treated by your doctor. Undiagnosed or untreated, these conditions spell disaster.

The Dead Swedish Patient

One example that vividly comes to mind is that of a Swedish tourist, forty-nine-year-old Kristoffer Andersson. Traveling with his wife and daughter, he was taking his first vacation in fifteen years. His sister, who lives in Florida, had spent months trying to get him to visit Orlando.

According to the details of the case, Kristoffer was a hothead, given to fits of anger. On the third day of the vacation, he got upset in a restaurant where the family was having breakfast. Kristoffer felt he was being overcharged for a soda. The incident escalated into a full-blown argument, and Kristoffer stormed out of the restaurant and decided to walk the nine miles back to the hotel. Forty-five minutes after leaving the restaurant, Kristoffer collapsed at a bus stop and fell to the ground. A witness called 911. Paramedics arrived and tried to revive him. But it was too late. Kristoffer died at the side of the road.

After they heard the agonizing news, the family became racked with guilt and blamed themselves for his death. They worried that the argument, coupled with the long walk back to the hotel, had done Kristoffer in.

For me, his death wasn't about blame or guilt. The real story could be told only through a full autopsy. Kristoffer was now my ward. As I looked him over, it was clear that he was overweight, by at least sixty pounds. There were no signs of external trauma from the fall, so I turned my attention to the internal examination. When someone keels over like he did, I look for the "big three": blood clots in the lungs, a heart problem, or a large bleed in the brain. This is a good way to start marking things off my list.

For starters, Kristoffer's lungs revealed that he was a smoker. They were streaked with black lines, but there was no evidence of clots. I ruled out the first of the three possible causes.

Next, I removed and weighed his heart. It was heavier than it should be—an indication of high blood pressure. I began to dissect it. As I sliced through Kristoffer's coronary arteries, I discovered what had killed him. There in my hands was the number one killer of men and women: a diseased heart. One of Kristoffer's coronary arteries was 95 percent blocked with a deadly amount of plaque. The artery was so narrow that only a trickle of blood was able to get through.

Starved for oxygen, his heart muscle became irritated, unable to beat normally. It started quivering, and when the heart starts quivering, it's not pumping. His heart stopped, dead.

At first, his family greeted my conclusion with disbelief. Kristoffer had never complained of chest pains or other symptoms that would suggest heart trouble. They thought he was as strong as an ox.

In truth, heart disease often goes undiagnosed. Thirty percent of people who die suddenly from a heart attack have had no prior symptoms. The heart attack is their first symptom.

But this knowledge did little to convince Kristoffer's family that their earlier argument and the walk didn't push him over the edge. Anger can certainly contribute to stress on your heart. But to have your heart go into an arrhythmia as his did, you must have a preexisting heart condition. Kristoffer had severe heart disease, and because it went untreated and undiagnosed for so long, it was inevitable that he would have a heart attack.

I spent time with his wife, daughter, and sister, drawing diagrams of what had happened to his heart and explaining the diagnosis as kindly as I could. As we talked, they told me that Kristoffer not only smoked heavily, he consumed several cans of soda a day, loved fast food, and never exercised—all of which played a role in his demise. A little preventive care on his part, including weight loss, would have gone a long way. Our discussions brought them sobering comfort, and they came to grips with the fact that he could have died anytime, anywhere. It was not their fault.

In the case of Kristoffer Andersson lies a vital message: If you're obese, you must put yourself under the care of a doctor. You want a doctor to detect abnormalities and treat you for them while you're alive, not a medical examiner to find them after you're dead.

> **TURN THE TABLES:** Prevent Deadly Diabetes Complications
>
> If you have diabetes and are overweight, shed just ten to fifteen pounds, and you can improve your health and help prevent some of the complications, such as heart, kidney, nerve, and eye disease.

Find a Diet You Can Live With

This is the tough part, and I like to use myself as an example of how tough it is. Coming from an Italian family where food was always within arm's reach, it seemed inevitable that I'd have a weight problem. I can't remember a meal that didn't have plates piled high with steaming spaghetti or lasagna and two types of red meat—after all, my dad was a butcher. My mom would even cook steaks just for our dogs because meat was so abundant in our household. As a kid and in my teens, I was chunky, and I felt unattractive. Today, I'd probably weigh three hundred pounds if I didn't watch it. To make matters worse, my first husband and his family were rail thin (no thrifty gene in their lineage); they could eat whatever they wanted and not gain an ounce. They'd have pancakes for breakfast, with coffee cake for dessert afterward. At 11 a.m., they'd pass out candy to everyone. It was hard for me to stay thin in that environment.

Nonetheless, I kept trying to lose weight, only to regain every pound I shed and then some. Every year I'd go up and down in weight. As I mentioned, after I gave birth to my oldest son, I put on loads of weight—forty pounds—and could not take it off. It's a myth that you lose weight while breast-feeding, because your body clings to the weight to have enough calories to nurse. Finally, I knew I had to do something. I joined a local weight-loss group, dropped that weight, and have kept it off. I got to know the nutritional value and calorie content of foods I ate. I largely gave up red meat, substituted whole wheat bread for regular bread (my downfall), and loaded up on fruits and vegetables. Then I started moving—mostly by running.

Sometimes figuring out what to eat for a healthy weight and a healthy body is like trying to piece together the clues of an autopsy. There are a lot of dead ends, and if one diet doesn't work, you find yourself back at square one. I don't advocate any particular diet—they all have their pros and cons. But what I think is the "perfect diet" is to become choosy about the foods you eat—not just for a couple of weeks or months but for the rest of your life. The perfect diet is not really a diet at all, but a way of eating you can live with every day.

Dietitians have a fairly good idea about how to do this, as well as plenty of solid evidence to back that up. As a rule, they tell us, we should eat lots of fruits and vegetables, favor whole grains over highly processed carbohydrates, and eat red meat sparingly. And we shouldn't eat any more than our body can handle.

That's where calorie counting comes in. Wait, don't skip this part. I'm not going to get tediously obsessive about this often-dreaded aspect of weight control. But whether you need to lose weight or you just want to keep the size you already have, you've got to know a little something about calories.

At its heart, the rule for losing weight is simple: Eat fewer calories than you burn. So it's a good idea to get familiar with the calorie count of foods. Just a couple of days of using a calorie-counting book, calculating the calories you consume, and writing them down can really help. You don't have to do this forever, just long enough to get a feel for it. To lose weight, the American Heart Association's rule of thumb is 1,200 to 1,500 calories a day for women, and 1,500 to 1,800 calories a day for men.

There are some easy ways to control calories without a lot of fuss. You can trick both your eyes and your stomach, for example. Use smaller dinner plates. Keep your servings in proportion. (No individual servings of food should be larger than your fist or the palm of your hand.) If you have a tendency to finish off a whole gallon of ice cream, try buying ice cream in single-serving ice cream bars or cups instead. To outsmart your hunger hormones, begin a couple of meals each week with a salad, piece of fresh fruit, or cup of broth-based soup. Each will help curb your appetite and automatically cut calories. Fruit and veggies, besides being nutritious and low in calories, are full of fiber and will make you feel full faster.

Get Moving

Exercise is important: Studies show that it staves off heart trouble, lowers blood pressure, normalizes blood sugar, strengthens bone health, improves depression and anxiety, and keeps your brain up to par as you age, among many other benefits. Extensive research has demonstrated that people who exercise even just a little bit tend to live longer. But many of us don't jog or do aerobics, don't walk when we can ride, don't move around when we can watch TV or play video games, and purposely avoid stairs when we can take the elevator. And to top that off, often to get in any exercise at all, we have to squeeze it into an already busy schedule—and I'm no exception.

My life is hectic in the morgue, and it's just as crazy when I get home. A dedicated medical examiner, I'm also a full-time mom and a wife. And just like every other mom and wife, I come home after work and make sure everything is in order with the household: I take care of the laundry, check in on my kids, and figure out what we're doing for dinner. Who has the energy to exercise? Well here's a tip: Trick yourself.

Here's what I do. I have a love/hate relationship with running, so I always say to myself, "I'll just go for a short walk. I'll listen to some good music, and it will help me relax." So I get my iPod and I start walking. And then I start walking a little faster. And then a great song comes on my iPod, and my blood starts pumping, and suddenly—I can run! I've done enough walking, and I can run! If I came home and said to myself, "I'll just straighten up, get dinner ready, and then go for a long run," I'd never do it. But by tricking myself into a smaller commitment, I can get started. And then it feels so good, I keep going.

I'm sure you've heard many of these ideas, but there's a reason I'll share them again: They work! I also try to find ways of making exercise an unavoidable part of my everyday life, so at work I take the stairs. When running errands, I gladly pick the farthest parking space out. Not only does it keep me walking, it saves my car from getting dented. There are plenty of ways to work exercise into your life: Play with your kids, garden and do yard work, walk briskly around the mall when you're shopping, walk your dog, clean your house, cook more meals at home, or go dancing. What you do will depend on your physical condition and what you most enjoy doing, but most people can get started with some simple shifts in these lifestyle activities or a walking program.

Try a Little Help from Weight-Loss Drugs

I believe medications for weight loss can be of help if you've tried everything to shed your excess weight, but without much success. Sometimes, a weight-loss medication is all you need to see some positive change and provide a little impetus. A caveat: That impetus won't go far, though, unless you make a sincere effort to follow the same old yada, yada, yada of dieting and exercise.

Diet drugs have come a long way from the days when certain pills were yanked from the market because they caused heart problems. Today, there are better, safer drugs. Two frontline drugs available for weight loss are Meridia (sibutramine), which controls eating by sending a signal of fullness to the brain so you're likely to eat less; and Xenical (orlistat) and its over-the-counter version

Alli, both of which block digestion of about 30 percent of the fat in your food. Xenical and Meridia typically help you lose anywhere from 5 to 10 percent of your body weight, but they do more than that: A recent study I read in the *British Journal of Medicine* reported that Xenical curbs diabetes, reduces harmful LDL cholesterol and blood pressure, and helps normalize blood sugar in people with diabetes. Meridia lowers triglycerides, a blood fat once thought relatively harmless but now considered dangerous.

Like any drugs, both have side effects, however. With Xenical, you have to follow a low-fat diet. If you don't, expect to experience loose, oily stools, since the excess fat that is blocked from absorption is quickly excreted. Meridia can sometimes raise your blood pressure, increasing the risk of heart attack or stroke.

While researching for this chapter, I learned that marijuana might be the future of weight loss. Well, okay, not exactly, but here's the scoop: As of this writing, there are new, hopefully about-to-be-approved diet drugs that block the brain's cannabinoid receptors, the same ones that are stimulated when smoking pot. Basically, these drugs would curb your "munchies," and they sound really promising.

I have a lot of faith in science, and I hope that more effective diet pills will be developed to help stem the tide of obesity. If you're someone with a serious weight problem and you have dangerous conditions like cholesterol or blood sugar problems along with it, don't be afraid to take the next step. Talk to your doctor about whether an obesity drug will help you.

Avoid weight-loss quackery, too. It's important to be smart about losing weight. I wouldn't recommend trying anything crazy, and there are plenty of crazy things out there, such as non-FDA-approved diet pills, herbs, and supplements that promise miraculous weight loss. We should all be careful about anything we put in our bodies, including dietary supplements.

So take it from a doctor who spends eight hours a day cutting up bodies in a morgue. There are lots of things you can do to avoid an unscheduled appointment with me—and losing weight in a healthy manner is one of them. Your life may depend on it.

Is Gastric Bypass Surgery for You?

Ten years ago, I would have never suggested that anyone consider weight-loss surgery. I believe it's a drastic measure. But according to recent research, the risks of morbid obesity are greater than the risks of surgery. You're a candidate if you have a BMI of 40 and higher, or a BMI of 35 and higher plus a serious weight-related illness such as diabetes or hypertension.

There are several types of weight-loss surgery, but the most common is gastric bypass. It involves stapling the stomach and forming a small pouch that can hold only about an ounce of food. Food goes into the pouch, then directly into the lower smaller intestine (the jejunum). The gastric bypass prevents your body from absorbing calories and makes your stomach so small that it's hard to eat too much. You'll feel full with as little as half a sandwich.

With gastric bypass surgery, you can lose quite a bit of weight, with a good chance of keeping it off. Weight-related conditions like diabetes, high blood pressure, high cholesterol, and sleep apnea often get better or disappear altogether. But you have to eat carefully, and you might have to take vitamin and mineral supplements to make up for deficiencies.

Like any surgery, weight-loss surgeries carry risks of infection, bleeding, blood clots, or reactions to anesthesia. There is the risk of death, too—a risk that depends on your age, general health, and any medical problems you have. The decision to have weight-loss surgery is something to talk to your doctor about. Honestly, if you're morbidly obese, you're likely to die from obesity or the complications of obesity. Given that possibility, I'd take my chances with the surgery.

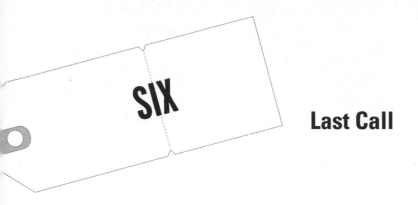

SIX

Last Call

Naked Rider

Her name was Lily Hammon, and she was found dead—and naked—in her driveway, leaving me to figure out whether it was a natural death, an accident, an injury, or something more sinister.

Back at work, I learned the details of the case from my investigators. At forty-one years old, Lily was a vibrant woman with a knack for telling jokes. She was a widow who had been living outside of town on an isolated ranch that provided a peaceful place for her favorite hobby—all-terrain vehicle (ATV) riding.

But the day of her death it was anything but peaceful. At about 12:30 p.m. on a sweltering hot day, her brother pulled into the driveway, ready to toss back a few beers with his sister. He spotted something odd. His heart sank at the sight. There on the ground, nude, was Lily.

When investigators arrived, they treated the area as a crime scene. They bagged her hands to preserve trace evidence in case there was foul play.

Information from Lily's devastated family came trickling in. They said she suffered from migraines. Occasionally associated with stroke, migraines can be triggered by food, chemicals, and bright lights. The family admitted that since her husband's death years ago from a heart attack, Lily had a proclivity to numb her grief with alcohol—and lots of it—throughout the day. That was an important clue to me, because when you drink large quantities of alcohol, sometimes you can end up with people you shouldn't be with and that can get you into trouble. If you're a woman, for example, and you drink to the point of intoxication, your risk of accidents and sexual assault is higher.

I also discovered that Lily had a bizarre habit: She liked to ride her ATV naked, ostensibly to work on her tan. The police officers working the case believed this habit may have contributed to her death, by possibly attracting unwanted, unsavory attention. Was Lily raped and murdered? The police were counting on me to answer those questions.

I carefully searched for evidence of rape, starting with her hands. I removed the bags to look for signs of a struggle. If someone tries to rape you, you're probably going to fight like crazy. Yet I could find no defensive injuries whatsoever. Nor were there tears or bruises on her genitalia. If Lily had been attacked, her assailant certainly didn't leave any visible clues. But a lack of evidence doesn't always mean no rape. Many times, especially if someone is high on drugs or alcohol, there may not be any injuries.

Next, I looked for the type of trauma most associated with deaths where sexual assault is involved: strangulation. I examined her neck for bruises. Unfortunately, Lily's body had already turned green and pink—the colors of decomposition—and it was impossible to identify bruises under those conditions. If Lily was strangled, I'd have to prove it in the internal examination.

After opening her chest cavity, I found that her internal organs were in surprisingly good shape, despite her years of alcohol abuse. There was one organ, though, with a hint of disease: her liver. It was tannish in color, not the normal healthy brown, and there was some scarring—all signs that meant early cirrhosis, the disease most closely associated with alcoholism. But the cirrhosis was not bad enough to cause her death.

Finding nothing else of note, I was left with one last body part to give me some answers: Lily's brain. I knew from the report that she had suffered from migraines. Were they truly migraines or something else, like a brain aneurysm, tumor, or recent head trauma? Examining the brain would answer those questions.

Once her skull was opened, I knew I had only a small window of time with which to work. In a decomposed body, the brain loses its shape very quickly. I had to get that initial look and I'd have to get it fast.

Any forensic pathologist will tell you that this part of an autopsy is particularly grisly for others to watch. An incision is made from ear to ear at the back of the head. The scalp is then folded back over the face to expose the skull, and the face turns into a ghastly mask. The morgue technician next turns on the bone saw to cut away the top of the head, and you hear the whine of blade cutting bone.

I managed to get a quick look at the exterior of Lily's brain. There was no blood, so that ruled out a burst aneurysm, a deadly fall, or a fatal blow from an assailant. She had no evidence of trauma at all. I took her brain out and held it in my gloved hands. It was like trying to hold toothpaste as it fell through my fingers. It would offer up no further clues.

One of the final steps in an autopsy is to focus on the neck to look for internal signs of strangulation. By the end of an autopsy, all the blood is drained from a body, giving me better visibility of the structures in the neck. The first place I look is the strap muscles of the neck for hemorrhage; there was none. The next place I look at is the hyoid bone, a small horseshoe-shaped bone in the neck that sits just under the jaw. Because the structure can be fractured by strangulation, a broken hyoid bone is a crucial finding in suspected cases of homicide. The hyoid bones in Lily's neck were intact, as was the thyroid cartilage in her neck, also vulnerable to strangulation. Lily was not strangled.

So far, the autopsy had revealed nothing.

My final hope for an answer would be in Lily's blood samples, but even those might lead nowhere. I might not be able to say how she died because toxicology on a decomposed body presents problems. The body starts releasing substances into the blood that normally aren't there, and the samples become corrupted.

The mystery of Lily's death weighed heavily on my mind. I kept my fingers crossed that the toxicology lab might find the answer. A few weeks passed and I received the report. At worst I expected a slate of inconclusive readings. But the report contained a surprising piece of evidence: Her blood was saturated with more than five times the legal definition of alcohol intoxication. I wasn't surprised to find the alcohol, but I was shocked by the amount. Lily had died of alcohol poisoning, also termed acute alcohol intoxication.

As a medical examiner, I've seen hundreds of people killed by the effects of alcohol. I get the people who, if at risk for suicide, will carry it out while they're intoxicated, since alcohol decreases inhibitions. I get the drunk drivers and the people they smash into. I get those who have suffered seizures or organ failure because of an alcohol addiction. Alcohol can kill in many different ways, and it keeps us busy in the morgue.

Lily, however, didn't die from the effects of alcohol on her behavior, or the long-term impact on her internal organs. She drank herself to death in a single sitting.

Alcohol is a drug. Like morphine or valium, it depresses the central nervous system and affects the body's most vital functions. Normally, your liver can process one drink—about four ounces of wine or one and a half ounces of hard liquor—in an hour. Blood alcohol concentration (BAC) is expressed in grams per deciliter. If you're drinking at a steady pace, by the time you reach about a 0.3 g/dl level, a marvelous defense mechanism kicks in to protect you from yourself: You fall asleep or pass out and can no longer drink. But if you consume too many drinks too quickly, the liver can't keep up with your intake. Blood alcohol skyrockets and begins depressing the central nervous system. Breathing slows and heart rate drops. Unless you receive urgent medical attention, you slip into a coma and may die.

That is exactly what happened to Lily Hammon. I ruled her death an accidental overdose. I don't think she meant to die.

Understandably, her family was devastated that Lily's drinking had taken such a fatal turn. But something good came from her death. After the tragedy, her brother—also an alcoholic—reached out for help by entering an alcohol rehab program, and this act brought great solace to the family.

It's always disheartening to see an otherwise healthy person land in my morgue, dead from alcohol abuse. Unfortunately, I see it all the time. Alcohol is the most commonly abused drug in the United States and in much of the world. According to the CDC, excessive alcohol use kills seventy-five thousand Americans a year, and it is the third-leading lifestyle-related cause of death in the country behind smoking and obesity.

There's nothing wrong with enjoying a drink or two responsibly on occasion. My husband, Mark, is a wine enthusiast, and we enjoy learning about wine and tasting selections from around the world. But our lives don't revolve around drinking.

Not being able to limit your alcohol consumption can morph into a serious problem. When you get addicted to alcohol, it affects your brain and your behavior. You ultimately lose control of the use of alcohol and you lose control of your life. Drinking is often the center of your life, even if there are bad consequences, such as problems with health, money, relationships, and performance at work or school.

Under the Influence: The Acute Effects of Alcohol

There are three major ways alcohol and many other drugs can kill you: acutely, chronically, and environmentally. By "acute," I mean a death that comes on fast, like Lily Hammon's alcohol poisoning, in which she died after a single bout of binge drinking. It can even kill you the first time you try it. I once autopsied a fourteen-year-old girl whose parents went out for the evening. Her older sister, who was supposed to be watching her, decided to go out with her boyfriend. With no supervision in the house, a bunch of other teens came over for a party and raided the parents' bar. The young girl, who had never had alcohol before, became very drunk. She died from alcohol poisoning. Deaths like this are relatively rare. I typically have only one to three a year come through my morgue, but even one is one too many.

When Drinking Gets Out of Hand: Chronic Effects of Alcohol Abuse

The damage from alcohol can also be done slowly and chronically over time but may still kill you, since most of the body's organs and systems are hit hard by heavy drinking. Not surprisingly, alcohol abusers suffer from a wide range of medical ills, including heart trouble, liver disease, and neurologic diseases. These are listed in the table on page 127.

Murder by Two-by-Four?

Damage to the liver in the form of cirrhosis is one of the most devastating chronic effects of alcohol and is often fatal. A few years ago, I had a case that seemed like an open-and-shut homicide but became less clear-cut as I delved deeper into the death investigation. Kyle Gilbert, a thirty-eight-year-old landscaper who lived with his mother, went to see a customer who was late paying his bill. Instead of cash, Kyle received an unexpected payment: He was ruthlessly beaten in the chest with a two-by-four. He eventually made it home only to shock his mother with his injuries. She wanted to call an ambulance, but Kyle preferred to nurse his wounds with a stiff drink.

Although his wounds healed slowly, he seemed to be on the road to recovery—until two weeks later. Kyle was sitting on his bed, talking to his mother, when he collapsed and stopped breathing. His mother called 911, and Kyle was rushed to the hospital by paramedics. Doctors said he showed signs of internal bleeding, possibly consistent with the beating he had received. Less than two hours after collapsing, Kyle was pronounced dead in the emergency room.

CHRONIC EFFECTS OF ALCOHOL ABUSE

Body Systems and Organs Affected	Complications
Nervous system	• Intoxication with drunkenness and coma • Withdrawal syndromes, sometimes with seizures or delirium tremens (DTs) • Brain wasting (dementia) • Nerve damage • Cerebellar degeneration (deterioration of the cerebellum, the area of the brain concerned with muscle coordination and balance)
Gastrointestinal	• Inflammation and irritation of the lining of the esophagus and stomach (esophagitis and gastritis) • Increased incidence of cancers of the mouth, pharynx, larynx, and esophagus • Liver damage, such as cirrhosis or alcoholic hepatitis • Inflammation of the pancreas (pancreatitis), sometimes leading to pancreatic failure, chronic diarrhea, and/or chronic pain
Cardiovascular	• Arrhythmia (irregular heartbeat) • Cardiomyopathy, a disease of the heart muscle causing an enlarged heart, which can lead to heart failure and death • Elevated fats in the bloodstream

Metabolic	• Low blood sugar
	• Lower than normal levels of potassium, magnesium, calcium, and phosphate in the blood
Endocrine	• Decreased testosterone
	• Testicular atrophy causing an increase in estrogen and thus the development of breast tissue in men (gynocomatia)
Skin	• Rosacea (you know this as W. C. Fields's nose)
	• Spider angiomas (harmless collections of small blood vessels under the skin often seen in men with liver failure from alcohol)
Blood	• Low platelets
	• Anemia
	• Risk of infection
	• Impaired blood clotting

Despite the two-week gap, both the police and my investigator saw a clear connection between the beating and Kyle's death. If the beating set off a chain of events that caused his death, even if the beating occurred two weeks or two years earlier, that's a homicide. To prove or disprove it, I conducted a complete autopsy.

For police, autopsies of possible homicide victims have a special urgency, because they can lead to arrests and potential prosecutions. But for me, they come with a unique burden. If the findings are inconclusive, the killers might go free, but if I make an incorrect diagnosis, the innocent might be blamed. With the investigation of a murder possibly brewing, police gathered in the morgue, awaiting answers from the autopsy.

As I began my investigation into the death, I noted in Kyle's medical records that he had cirrhosis of the liver from alcoholism. As I began the external exam, I noticed that Kyle's skin was jaundiced, a sign of liver disease. But what really attracted my attention was the incredible bruising on his body. He was covered with more than a dozen bruises, still painfully visible after two weeks.

I found one wound particularly alarming. It was just above the costal margin, the bottom of the rib cage, and was seven inches long and three inches wide, a haunting imprint of a two-by-four. I had to wonder: Did the blow injure his aorta? His liver? His small intestine? How bad was it?

A violent blunt force to the body such as slamming into a steering wheel or receiving a blow from a two-by-four can cause fatal internal bleeding. When this occurs, blood seeps out of the damaged organ or vessel and pools inside the abdominal cavity. Though unusual, an internal injury like this may not bleed until days after the trauma.

Kyle's external examination was dramatic: He was bleeding from his nose, mouth, and even from his rectum. All signs still pointed to murder. But to unravel the mystery of the bleeding, I had to delve inside Kyle's body.

Once I made the Y incision and removed the chest plate, I carefully inspected the flesh beneath the most vicious bruise on Kyle's body. As I suspected, this single devastating blow had caused damage deep in the abdominal wall musculature. If I found pooling of blood inside the abdominal cavity, I'd have my smoking gun.

But then I got my first big surprise of the autopsy. I found no blood pooling in his abdominal cavity or his pleural cavity. With the exception of the deep bruising, I couldn't find any internal damage from the two-by-four at all. I was unable to find the concrete internal evidence to prove murder. Without this, the police couldn't arrest the man who had beaten Kyle for murder.

If Kyle did not die from the intense beating, then what killed him? And what caused him to cough up blood? I continued to look internally for reasons that might have contributed to his demise. I knew that Kyle had suffered from cirrhosis of the liver. Nevertheless, the condition of his liver was worse than I expected. Normally, a liver has a beautiful smooth capsule and is brown with very sharp edges. His was gnarly and yellow, as if studded with kernels of corn.

Cirrhosis is a liver disease most closely associated with viral hepatitis or, as in Kyle's case, alcoholism. But liver problems don't typically lead to sudden death.

Liver cirrhosis typically develops over the course of a decade or more. As liver cells die and are replaced by fibrous scar tissue, the organ begins to fail. Toxins accumulate in the blood, resulting in problems that range from nausea to coma. Eventually, scar tissue overtakes the liver, turning it into a mass of fibrous nodules. Kyle had what is called "end-stage cirrhosis." Even so, the advanced cirrhosis still didn't explain his death. People can have liver cirrhosis at autopsy, but it doesn't mean they died from it. So far, there was no definitive evidence that Kyle had died from his liver disease.

I had to move on to other organs in search of a cause of death. Maybe he had a heart attack; I didn't know. But upon examining Kyle's heart, I saw nothing out of the ordinary. Then after opening his stomach, I made a startling discovery. He had enough blood in there to fill a liter-sized Coke bottle, and it distended his stomach. The average adult needs about five liters of blood to live, and Kyle had bled out at least a full liter. Could this have somehow stemmed from his earlier beating?

I examined the remainder of his gastrointestinal tract. His intestines contained more blood, but there was no indication of the source. Next, I moved upward to where the esophagus enters the stomach. It was there that I finally found what I was looking for: an enlarged blood vessel that had recently burst.

As it turned out, varicose veins called "varices" had formed on Kyle's esophagus. They are caused by liver disease and are similar to the wiggly, dilated varicose veins that some people have in their legs. The walls of esophageal varicose veins are very thin and prone to rupturing.

Varices are formed when the scarring of cirrhosis slows the flow of blood through the liver. This causes blood to back up in the portal vein, which delivers blood from the stomach and intestines to the liver. This condition is called portal hypertension. Blood has such a difficult time getting through a scarred liver that it bypasses the organ, taking other veins up and around the base of the esophagus to get back to the heart. These veins expand beyond their normal capacity, turning into varices with dangerously thin walls. Because the blood pressure inside the varices is higher than inside normal blood vessels, and the walls of the vessels are thin, they burst easily and can bleed profusely. Ninety percent of people with cirrhosis of the liver will develop esophageal varices; 30 percent of them will eventually bleed from the varices. The death rate from bleeding esophageal varices, even the first time it happens, is between 33 and 50 percent.

Only one question remained: Did the beating contribute to the rupturing of the blood vessels, or was the timing sheer coincidence?

I couldn't connect the beating to his bleeding varices. In retracing the chain of events that led to Kyle Gilbert's untimely death, the initiating event in this case was chronic alcoholism that led to cirrhosis of the liver. The final, frightening episode in Kyle's life was a massive hemorrhage from ruptured varices in his esophagus.

With that diagnosis, I called the police to tell them that my autopsy results showed that the cause of death wasn't related to a criminal offense, and the man who beat him was not responsible for his death.

In forensic pathology, the manner of death is limited to one of five categories: homicide, suicide, accident, natural, and undetermined. By convention, in most medical examiners' offices, when someone dies from the acute effects of alcohol (like alcohol poisoning), we call those deaths accidents. When someone dies from the chronic effects of drinking (like bleeding to death from esophageal varices brought on by liver failure), we call those deaths natural. Deaths from abuse of alcohol don't fit neatly into our five choices of accident, homicide, natural, suicide, or undetermined.

Deadly Withdrawal

A problem that distinguishes alcohol from many other drugs is how physiologically addicting it is. When someone stops drinking after long-term use, he or she may experience "alcohol withdrawal syndrome." It is triggered when the central nervous system attempts to adjust to the sudden absence of alcohol in the body.

Symptoms include mild tremors, which can kick in as swiftly as six hours after you stop drinking; seizures, which can be fatal in chronic alcoholics who have stopped drinking; or delirium tremors (DTs), characterized by confusion, disorientation, delusion, hallucinations, and agitation. DTs occur about forty-eight to seventy-two hours after drinking has stopped. Though the rarest of withdrawal symptoms, DTs can progress to cardiovascular collapse or death. With a severe dependency, withdrawal from alcohol can kill you—which is why stopping drinking after chronic alcohol abuse is best done in a supervised facility. Some alcoholics need to be observed in a hospital while they try to stop drinking. One of my sadder cases was of an alcoholic who quit cold turkey to try and win back his ex-wife, who had divorced him because of his drinking. He suffered a fatal seizure when his brain went into withdrawal. His body was so used to living with alcohol that it couldn't function without it.

Don't Be Dumb About Drinking: Environmental Effects of Alcohol

When I use the term "environmental deaths," I mean encounters or situations related to alcohol or drug use that put you in jeopardy, such as loss of life while driving under the influence. Alcohol is a leading cause of highway deaths. Forty-one percent of all traffic fatalities involve alcohol. Suicides are heavily influenced by alcohol, which by lowering inhibitions can lead to a spur-of-the-moment self-killing. Even at the lowest measurable level, alcohol affects your perception, judgment, reaction time, information processing, learning, hearing, and peripheral vision. When you're drunk, you don't even know how impaired you are, and this lack of awareness can result in all sorts of accidents, from the unimaginable to the bizarre.

Burning Questions

I listen to the radio during my morning commute to work. One summer morning I heard on the radio that there was a car fire in one of the parking garages in downtown Orlando, and a dead body was found in the burning car. I knew I would see that body when I got to work. Sure enough, it was my first case of the day.

Several hours earlier, at about 4 a.m., a parking lot attendant had spotted a car with its engine running. In the passenger seat was a man apparently sleeping. He did not wake the occupant, however, but returned to his office instead. A half hour later, he got the shock of his life. The man's car was engulfed in flames and the horrified attendant couldn't even get near the vehicle. He called 911, and the dispatcher told him to pull the fire alarm.

Arriving on the scene, the Orlando Fire Department quickly put out the fire. When the smoke cleared, investigators got their first clear look at what is a most uncommon sight—a fire death in a parked car. Less than 2 percent of all auto fires result in a death, and most of these deaths occur as a result of crashes. The reason? When a car fire starts, an able-bodied person stuck inside will usually get out before being burned.

Because the driver did not exit in time, investigators thought he was already dead before the fire started or something or someone must have kept him there against his will. It is not uncommon for the body of a homicide victim to be burned in order to hide evidence and thwart the investigation.

So was it a homicide or an accident? Within an hour, a team of detectives and arson specialists arrived to investigate. They looked at the exterior of the car, the parking garage, and the area around it. They didn't want to do anything to the body, for fear of destroying any evidence that I might find. Because of the fire's mysterious circumstances, foul play was strongly suspected.

One of the first priorities in the case of a fire victim is to determine the victim's physical condition at the moment the fire began. Was he alive or dead when the fire started? If he was alive, was he injured or perhaps shot?

Because it is nearly impossible to detect any external injuries or gunshot wounds on charred remains, I x-rayed the victim. I then examined the developed film, and before making even a single incision, I could already draw one tentative conclusion. On the X-rays there appeared to be no sign of trauma that could have led to the victim's death before the fire. The only injuries I could see on the film were those he sustained during the blaze.

During the external exam, one of my first tasks was to identify the body's unique burn pattern. Burn patterns can confirm whether the victim was motionless when the fire burned. The back, buttocks, and back of the legs were not as charred as the rest of his body because they were up against the seat, and there was less oxygen getting to those areas. The lack of burning in these areas proved the victim didn't move after the car caught on fire—another possible indication that he may have been dead before the fire started.

In burn cases, there are specific parts of the body that can reveal even stronger indicators of when a person died—the nose and mouth. I wanted to find out if he was breathing in the products of combustion, such as soot, as the car became engulfed in flames. If I found no soot, it would be strong evidence that the victim was not alive. There was soot in his mouth and nose, which was important but not conclusive. The soot could simply mean that the smoke from the intensely contained fire had drifted into the open cavities.

The only way I could know for sure was to inspect the respiratory tract from the inside. I began with the Y incision, and after opening the rib cage, I found that for the most part the victim's internal organs were not affected by the heat.

I took fluid samples from the victim for toxicology tests and then began my search inside the body's cavity. Because the death was a suspected homicide, I looked for any signs of foul play or trauma that could not been seen on the X-rays, such as internal bleeding or perhaps even strangulation. But here, too, I found nothing out of the ordinary and no sign of injuries indicating that the victim may have been restrained.

Next, I opened the respiratory tract. Within seconds, I uncovered something that contradicted almost every previous assumption in the case. There was soot deep in the victim's trachea and all the way down into his lung tissue. This finding was undeniable proof that the victim had been alive when the fire started. Without a doubt, he was breathing sooty material.

Through testing to reveal carbon monoxide in his system, my autopsy revealed that this poisonous gas had displaced nearly 75 percent of the oxygen in his blood. My original hypothesis that he was dead before flames engulfed his car was shattered by these findings, and I determined that he died from smoke inhalation from the fire.

What I still didn't know was the manner of death. Was it a homicide?

While I waited for the results of the arson investigation and the toxicology report, the homicide detectives uncovered another lead. A cell phone was salvaged from the wreckage and police were able to identify the victim through phone records. They immediately contacted his family. The victim's name was Carlos Martin. He had just started a new job as a marketing consultant and had been out at a party with some of his college fraternity brothers who lived in the Orlando area. It wasn't much, but at least I knew who the victim was and some of the circumstances that led up to his death.

I felt terrible for his mother and aunt, who came here from New York City. No one would tell them anything definitive while the case was investigated for homicide, and it was heart wrenching. They just wanted the truth, and I assured them that I would try to give them answers as best I could.

It took several more months for the preliminary results of the arson investigation to arrive. The point of origin was somewhere in the driver's seat near the dash, but although three experienced investigators and sets of engineers examined the car three separate times, they couldn't come up with a definitive cause. They were fairly certain, however, that the fire was not set by any person, including Carlos.

Although I may never know how the fire began, I hoped that the toxicology report would shed light on the other remaining mystery. Why didn't Carlos get out of the car once it started burning?

I began wondering if he had overdosed on an illicit drug. It was an implication that Carlo's family denied emphatically. Their son did not use drugs.

In this case, toxicology tests proved that Carlo's family was right. He had not used any illicit substances the night of his death, but he did, apparently, drink quite a bit of alcohol. He was very intoxicated. There was slightly over .2 g/dl of alcohol in his blood. The legal limit is .08—he was 150 percent higher than that—which should give you an idea of how intoxicated he was. With the toxicology report in hand, I knew why Carlos did not get out of that fire.

After a long day of business meetings, Carlos Martin went out for drinks with friends. He didn't drink alcohol very often. By the time he left the bar, Carlos's blood alcohol level was very high, over twice the legal limit. In the garage, Carlos started the ignition and turned the air on to keep him cool on a hot Orlando evening, but he quickly realized he was too drunk to drive. He then did what many would consider prudent. He put the car in park and decided to sleep it off on the passenger side of the car where he'd be more comfortable.

Within a half hour, a fire broke out somewhere under the dash. The fire quickly engulfed the passenger side, where Carlos was sleeping. Because he had excessive alcohol in his system and he was not usually a heavy drinker, Carlos remained unconscious. The fire consumed the vehicle and Carlos along with it.

Although the freak accident was difficult for Carlos's family to bear, one of my findings brought some relief. He died fairly quickly, most likely from the inhalation injuries. But death, no matter what the circumstances, always leaves survivors with the same difficult question—why did it have to happen?

How Not to Die from Alcohol Abuse

Maybe you've found yourself drinking too much or using more alcohol than you intended. Maybe you've had an accident or a social or legal problem caused by your alcohol use. Or maybe you have loved ones who are worried about your drinking. Experts have set guidelines that can help you determine if you have a problem, and these are summarized in the quiz on page 137. Use it to do a reality check to ascertain if alcohol is taking over your life.

With alcohol, drinking more than four drinks per occasion, or fourteen in a week, is considered "hazardous drinking" for men. Women who have more than three drinks per occasion, or seven in a week, fall into this category, too. If

> ## Do You Have a Drinking Problem?
>
> Answer the following four questions to help you find out if you or someone close to you has a drinking problem.
>
> - Have you ever felt you should cut down on your drinking?
> - Have people annoyed you by criticizing your drinking?
> - Have you ever felt bad or guilty about your drinking?
> - Have you ever had a drink first thing in the morning to steady your nerves or to get rid of a hangover?
>
> One "yes" answer suggests a possible alcohol problem. If you responded yes to more than one question, it is very likely that you have a problem with alcohol. In either case, it is important that you see your physician right away to discuss your responses to these questions.
>
> Even if you answered no to all of the above questions, if you are having drinking-related problems with your job, relationships, health, or with the law, you should seek help.
>
> Source: The National Institute on Alcohol Abuse and Alcoholism (NIAAA)

you're a "hazardous drinker," try to reduce your alcohol consumption or quit altogether.

Cut Back On Your Drinking

Some drink-reducing strategies I recommend include having a drink of water or soda between alcoholic drinks; limiting yourself to only a few drinks a week; or making a contract with yourself to drink only on planned days and time periods. Try taking a break from alcohol for a week if you're a heavy drinker and see how you feel physically and emotionally. When you succeed and feel better, you may find it easier to cut down for good. Watch out for people, places, or times that make you drink, even if you do not want to. Stay away from people who drink a lot or bars where you used to go. Plan ahead of time what you will do to avoid drinking when you are tempted.

Help with a drinking problem should come first from a doctor, since addic-

> **TURN THE TABLES**: Avoid Emotional Drinking
>
> Don't drink when you're angry or upset or have had a bad day. This is a habit you need to break if you want to drink less. If you find you can't do this on your own, you need additional help.

tion is a life-shattering medical problem. Your doctor can give you support and help you find a treatment program that fits your needs. Your doctor can also treat withdrawal symptoms and other alcohol-related problems.

Try Antialcohol Medications

In addition, there are now three FDA-approved medications that can be prescribed by your doctor to help you quit drinking and avoid a relapse:

- Campral (acamprosate) is thought to restore the normal brain balance, which has been disturbed in someone who is alcohol dependent.
- Revia or Depade tablets or the injectable Vivitrol (naltrexone) may help you drink less by decreasing your craving for alcohol.
- Antabuse (disulfiram) will prevent you from drinking. Drinking even a very small amount of alcohol will make you nauseous and possibly lead to vomiting. Of the three medications, this is the only one that will make you feel sick.

Seek Counseling

Medications alone will not solve an alcohol problem. In fact, one of the most hopeful messages coming out of current research is that the brain abnormalities associated with addiction to alcohol can be reversed through counseling. For that reason, all sorts of psychosocial interventions, ranging from psychotherapy to 12-step programs, can and do help. Therapy, either individually or in a group, can supply you with coping skills (such as exercising after work instead of going to a bar), and appears to hold particular promise. Other ways of treating alcohol problems include inpatient rehab, usually running a month or more; or outpatient treatment, done under the supervision of doctors and psychologists.

Build Support

Another vital step is to build a network of supportive people while breaking away from friends who are still drinking. The urge to drink is hard to resist

---

LIFE LESSONS: A Sensible Drinking Limit

If you don't have a problem with alcohol, it's probably safe for you to enjoy a moderate amount without injuring your health. Moderate drinking, in fact, may protect against heart disease and stroke. A moderate, sensible drinking limit for people who don't have a problem with alcohol is:

- For men, no more than two drinks per day.
- For women, no more than one drink per day.
- For people over sixty-five years old, no more than one drink per day.

when you're with your drinking buddies and watching them imbibe. To avoid these temptations, surround yourself with healthy, helpful nondrinkers instead.

I urge people who abuse alcohol to try to stop and to replace the drinking with a healthy activity. Breaking a drinking habit is never easy, but alcohol is not the answer. As long as you think it is, you take the risk that somebody like me may see you dead.

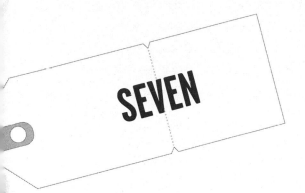

SEVEN

Dying to Get High

A Deadly Combination

At age twenty-nine, Tony Solito had all the trappings of a good life, from a well-paying job to a lovely home in suburbia. His life was rich in less material ways, as well: Family photos and home videos show him as a loving husband and father of two beautiful little girls.

But there are pictures missing here—of a secretive life that brought him to rest on a stainless steel autopsy table in my morgue one summer morning.

Tony Solito's journey to the morgue began the previous evening. Coming off a long, hard day at work, he made plans to go out drinking with his buddies, despite the objections of his wife, Sandra. Tony was a diabetic, and she was rightly worried about the effects of alcohol on his diabetes. Tony assured his wife that he wouldn't be out late and that he would be fine.

Yet when Tony got home at around 4 a.m., he was incoherent and seemed drunk. The next morning, his daughters bounded into the living room to wake up their father, but he was unresponsive and cold to the touch. Panicked, Tony's wife called 911. Paramedics soon arrived and tried to revive him but their efforts were in vain. Tony Solito was already dead.

Sandra was convinced that his heavy drinking, combined with his diabetes, was responsible for his death. Overcome with guilt, she wondered whether she could have saved her husband had she tried harder to keep him home. She knew all too well that consuming large amounts of alcohol could be extremely harmful for Tony. Diabetics like Tony should drink alcohol sparingly, since too much can dangerously lower or elevate blood sugar.

Tony, like many diabetics, had to undergo a daily regimen of injections to survive. But he had not given his condition the attention it deserved. From reading his medical records, I knew that he didn't take care of himself, he didn't eat well, and his blood sugar was always very high—situations that concerned his doctor. Clearly, Tony had very poorly controlled diabetes, and that can really do a number on a body.

With these facts in hand, I began the external examination, thinking about the ways in which diabetes could have caused his death. One way could be a condition known as ketoacidosis, which can be brought on by alcohol intoxication in an insulin-dependent diabetic like Tony. Ketoacidosis begins with a high blood sugar level, technically known as hyperglycemia. Hyperglycemia comes about if and when there is inadequate insulin circulating to escort blood sugar into cells. Desperate for a source of energy, the body begins burning fat instead of glucose as fuel. Fat then breaks down into acids known as ketones, which can be toxic if allowed to accumulate in the blood. If enough ketones build up, they cause ketoacidosis. Its symptoms include nausea, vomiting, tiredness, frequent urination, and a fruity odor to the breath. Anyone with these symptoms should seek help immediately because, if not caught quickly, a person can become quite sick and may end up dying.

If I found both ketones and a high glucose level in Tony's body, I would be almost certain that ketoacidosis took his life. Hypoglycemia, on the other hand, is harder to detect postmortem, since glucose levels drop after death. To answer this question I collected eye fluid from his eyes, which correlates with blood glucose levels.

The toxicology lab would also test Tony's blood alcohol level and perform a general toxicology screen. As is routine, I'd have to wait weeks for the lab results.

As I viewed the body, I looked for needle tracks and signs of trauma, but I didn't see anything. His external examination was pretty benign. I hoped that the internal exam would give more clues so that I could provide some answers to Tony's grieving widow.

After opening him up and dissecting his internal organs, I checked his heart for atherosclerosis or coronary artery disease, because it's so prevalent in people with diabetes, even in someone as young as Tony. Atherosclerosis occurs when plaque accumulates inside the coronary arteries, restricting the flow of blood. Diabetes creates an environment that gives rise to this blood vessel disease as elevated glucose attaches to chemicals in the walls of blood vessels, a process that promotes the formation of plaque and causes the blood vessels to narrow. Surprisingly, Tony had no atherosclerosis, even though he was a terribly uncontrolled diabetic.

There were other abnormalities, however: an enlarged heart, a sign of high blood pressure that could lead to arrhythmias; a very enlarged, round, and fatty liver—the telltale signs of either diabetes or heavy drinking; and heavy, fluid-filled lungs, which told me that Tony had lingered in a coma before he died. A terminal coma typically causes the lungs to fill up with fluid. I now knew he did not die suddenly from an arrhythmia.

Unlike television shows like *CSI,* we do not solve our cases in an hour. The real thing takes longer. I usually have to wait weeks for key pieces of evidence like toxicology reports before I can close a case. When the toxicology report on Tony Solito finally arrived, it turned the case upside down. There was surprise after surprise, and I was totally unprepared for what I read. To start with, there was no alcohol in his blood at all. Tony did not drink himself to death.

Next, I flipped through the report to find Tony's ketone and sugar analysis. Again, I was shocked by what I did not find: There were no ketones. He did have elevated glucose—200 mg/dl—but that wasn't high enough to kill him. I crossed ketoacidosis off the list of possible causes of death, as well as death from low blood sugar.

My final surprise on the report was the unmasking of Tony's killer: a lethal combination of heroin and cocaine. He had not gone out drinking with his buddies; he was out using drugs with his buddies, and I mean hard-core drugs in levels high enough to kill. The heroin level by itself was lethal, and the cocaine only further irritated his heart, possibly finishing the job and causing it to stop beating completely. Bottom line: Tony Solito died of heroin and cocaine intoxication.

The news came as a shock to Tony's wife. Although she realized that his drinking did not kill him, the full extent of his recklessness was difficult to accept. I see many deaths like this that are senseless and cruel, but in some cases when death seems so avoidable, I can only wonder what causes people to make such bad decisions. This guy needed a slap across the face and to be shaken into taking care of himself. Once you have children, at the very least, get your life together and live responsibly enough to take care of your family. Dying from drugs when you have a family leaves a tragic legacy, and watching this happen is one of the saddest parts of my work.

The lesson in Tony Solito's story is this: A man's life ended in a tragic and unnecessary way. As much as the heroin and cocaine, his refusal to take charge of his own health led to his premature death. In that tragedy, Tony is not unique.

I often ask myself why anyone would use illegal drugs. I'm sure there are many reasons. I suppose you might feel you're missing something in your life, and you use the drug to numb your negative emotions or as a substitute for whatever is missing. And I guess you could use drugs a few times to see what it's like; it makes you feel good, so you keep using it. By that time, you're hooked, and nothing else matters but getting more drugs. My patients can't tell me why they used drugs; I just see the tragic results of their decisions.

Whenever I autopsy someone who used drugs or was hooked on them, I think of a guy named James Connor, a young professional who was supposedly happy and successful until he got addicted to cocaine. James went from being a handsome, muscular, athletic man with a beautiful smile to a thin, disheveled, unemployed, mostly toothless shell of his former self. I met him not because he died, but because his elderly father had died.

James had been living with his father, who just happened to die from a heart attack while sitting in a lounge chair. Instead of reporting the death to authorities, James kept putting covers and tarps over his father's badly decomposing body. The house had the stench of every rotting thing you might call to mind. Yet James chose to live with it so he could continue to collect his father's retirement checks to buy more drugs. That is addiction.

The effects of drug abuse and addiction are specifically tied to the type of substance. Among illicit drugs, the big two for me in the morgue are still cocaine and heroin.

Killer Cocaine

Cocaine, the glamour dust of the late seventies, is the most commonly abused illicit drug we encounter in the morgue. Derived from the coca plant, cocaine was used for centuries by South American Indians who chewed the leaves for its stimulant properties, and since 1884 as medicine in a local anesthetic. According to the 2006 National Survey of Drug Use and Health, approximately 35.3 million Americans aged twelve and older have tried cocaine at least once in their lifetimes, and it is believed that hundreds of millions of people use cocaine worldwide.

Who uses cocaine? We often hear that it is used by the privileged, the successful, and the professional. But I have seen people from all walks of life do cocaine, rich or poor—and die from it. Teenagers are frequent users, and the elderly have come through my morgue, dead from cocaine. There are no clear connections between cocaine use and education, occupation, or socioeconomic status.

Cocaine can be snorted, injected, or smoked depending on its form. Powder cocaine is snorted or injected. Crack is simply powder cocaine mixed with baking soda and water, then heated and allowed to harden into rocks to create a smokable drug. Smoking crack cocaine produces such an overwhelming but brief rush that it can trigger a relentless craving.

It doesn't matter which form you use; all forms can do you in—and do it in many different ways. Unlike alcohol and heroin, as well as other narcotics, all of which are central nervous system depressants, cocaine is a stimulant. It works by triggering the release of catecholamines (chemicals in the body that play a role in its response to a stress), blocking their reabsorption by the nerves and thus prolonging their action in the body. This situation spikes your blood pressure, quickens your heart rate, churns out more blood sugar, and heats up your body temperature.

Cocaine is best known for its powerful mental kick, but blood vessels take the hardest beating. Cocaine-triggered strokes and heart attacks—both of which can occur in people with no known cardiovascular disease—are quite common, caused by the sudden elevation of blood pressure and spasms of blood vessels. The damage can come on suddenly and acutely, even with the very first use of the drug or unexpectedly thereafter. Cocaine can also induce seizures. Chronic cocaine use has also been found to accelerate atherosclerosis, plaque inside the vessels of the heart that constrict blood flow and makes each subsequent use of cocaine more dangerous for the heart. I've listed other killer consequences in the table on page 147.

It's dangerous to use cocaine under any circumstances, but if you have pre-existing heart disease, high blood pressure, or any medical condition, you're making a date with the Grim Reaper. Early in my career, while I was working in Miami, Florida, I autopsied a sixty-two-year-old cabaret performer who was found dead at the makeup table in his dressing room during intermission. He had a history of high blood pressure, and died from a dissected aorta, commonly seen with hypertension. Although the walls of the aorta have a degree of elasticity, a rise in blood pressure can partially tear the aortic walls if they are weakened by cardiovascular disease. Blood then dissects, or cuts down, the wall of the aorta, causing it to rupture. I did my routine toxicology testing, not expecting to find anything but a little alcohol. I thought it would be a natural death, until I found out from the toxicology report that he was high on cocaine. The cocaine jacked up his blood pressure and precipitated the aortic dissection

DEADLY DANGERS OF COCAINE USE

Body Systems and Organs Affected	Complications
Cardiovascular	Sudden cardiac death with as little at 20 mg; heart attack, rupture of the aorta, irregularities in the heart's rhythm, cardiomyopathy (disease of the heart muscle), high blood pressure
Neurological	Stroke, inflammation of blood vessels in the brain, headache, bleeding in the brain, seizures, and partial or complete loss of consciousness
Pulmonary	Chronic cough, lung irritation, collapsed lungs, pulmonary edema or hemorrhage, lung inflammation
Ear, nose, and throat	Hoarseness, destruction of nasal structures, colds, and sinusitis
Psychiatric	Anxiety, agitation, delirium, paranoia, suicide, severe depression, violent behavior
Infectious complications	AIDS (via contaminated needles), endocarditis (bacterial infection of the heart valves), tetanus, viral hepatitis due to IV use
Other	Hyperthermia (unusually high body temperature), muscle injury, kidney failure, intermittent loss of feeling in the extremities, tremors, intestinal ischemia (death of part of the intestine due to loss of blood)

and his death. I ruled the case accidental, since the cocaine contributed to bringing on his death.

Many drugs are "dose dependent," meaning the higher the dose, the more pronounced the effects. Cocaine, however, is not dose dependent. You never know how much, or how little, will kill you—which is why doing cocaine is like playing Russian roulette. I once had a case involving two brothers who used cocaine frequently. Just after snorting some cocaine, one of the brothers had a seizure and died, while the other brother looked on. When I spoke to the surviving brother, he just wouldn't believe that cocaine had killed his brother. His rationale was that he had used the exact same amount at the same time from the same source. That's the scary part of cocaine. It can kill you after the first time, the second time, or hundredth time you use it. If you don't want to take a chance on dying prematurely, I suggest you do not go anywhere near cocaine.

Heroin: Mainline to Death

Heroin is processed from naturally occurring morphine, a derivative of the opium poppy, and usually appears as a white or brown powder. Approximately 3.8 million Americans aged twelve or older reported trying heroin at least once during their lifetimes, reports the 2006 National Survey on Drug Use and Health. This report also indicated that there were 91,000 persons aged twelve or older who had used heroin for the first time within a recent twelve-month period.

Heroin is a powerfully addictive drug that produces short-term feelings of euphoria and relaxation. Highly addictive, heroin frequently hooks users for the rest of their lives, unless it simply kills them first. Death usually comes by overdose.

Unlike cocaine, heroin is dose dependent. When you're using heroin regularly, you develop a tolerance to the drug. Once this happens, you must have more heroin to achieve the same intensity or effect you're seeking—a development that's the first step on the road to addiction. If you stop taking heroin for a short period of time—say, during a stint in jail—but then resume your "normal" dose, you can die because you've lost your tolerance to the drug. That normal dose is now an overdose. I typically suspect a heroin overdose when someone is found dead in a public bathroom, alley, or other place, with no apparent trauma, especially after I learn from my investigators that the victim was released from jail twenty-four hours earlier.

Users administer heroin in several ways, including snorting and injecting, and they may inhale its vapors when heated (called chasing the dragon). Some mix heroin with cocaine in a "speedball" that is usually injected intravenously or smoked, producing a more intense rush than heroin alone. This is dangerous because the combination of a stimulant (cocaine) with a depressant (heroin) increases the risk of death with one or both drugs. I've seen plenty of people poison themselves to death like this.

In addition to the effects of the drug itself, if you inject yourself, you risk contracting infectious diseases such as HIV/AIDS or hepatitis from contaminated needles. Heroin bought off the street is often cut with various substances such as sugar or other dilutants, causing an added danger. It's also common to cut heroin with talcum powder. When both get injected into the vein, the heroin eventually gets metabolized and excreted, while the talcum powder is filtered out in the lungs. Because talcum powder is a foreign substance, it causes scar tissue to build up in the lungs. Chronic intravenous heroin users, if they live that long, can die from not being able to breathe due to this scar tissue. Because heroin abusers don't know the actual strength of the drug or its true contents, they're at a great risk of overdosing or dying. Overdose can also spring from an uncut batch that is very pure.

An Inconvenient Death

Like most drugs, heroin puts you in bad company. Thirty-year-old Nancy Lugar, mother of two, is a case in point. Early one weekday morning, she was found by a bicyclist, facedown in a grassy drainage ditch next to a railroad track. Two days prior, her husband, Michael, had driven her to her job as a waitress at an

DEADLY DANGERS OF HEROIN USE

Drowsiness, sedation, confusion

Respiratory depression, death due to overdose

HIV/AIDS, hepatitis A, hepatitis B, hepatitis C, bacterial infections, including tetanus and botulism

Chronic lung disease

Orlando restaurant. But according to police, she never made it to work. Michael also told us that Nancy was a recovering heroin addict. It was a really sad story to me. He knew she had a drug problem, and he wanted to save her.

One of the important clues I uncovered in the external examination was that she had linear scars in the front nook of her elbow—the part where your arm bends and where blood is drawn. This is also a site where heroin is commonly injected. Some of the scars were old and confirmed Nancy's known history of IV drug abuse. But there was evidence of recent use as well. She had a fresh needle mark in her left arm.

As is customary, my morgue technician then took urine samples from her bladder and blood samples from the artery in her leg to be sent to the toxicology lab.

Several weeks later, when the toxicology report came in, the first findings were no surprise to me. High levels of morphine were present in her blood, meaning she was probably on heroin. Morphine is a pain medication, but it is also the breakdown product of heroin. But surprisingly, the lab found another drug in high levels in Nancy's blood: the powerful stimulant cocaine. Like Tony Solito, she had succumbed to a fatal drug intoxication.

On the morning of her death, Nancy's husband dropped her off at her job, but instead of going to work, she went to a nearby house and injected herself with a mixture of cocaine and heroin. She got the high she craved, but then the powerful drug combination began to take its deadly toll. She went into a coma, and the other drug users there probably thought she was sleeping it off. But Nancy was not asleep. She was dead.

Left with a dead woman in a house full of drugs, and not wanting to draw the attention of authorities, Nancy's fellow users faced a grim dilemma: what to do with the body? They came up with a heartless solution to this inconvenient death: Toss it in a ditch. And that's exactly what they did.

The people you hang out with when you do drugs are not the nicest people in the world. They don't care about you or what happens to you. They will dump you like a piece of trash.

The Scary New Drug Addiction

I'm seeing more and more people self-destruct these days due to prescription drug abuse. And it's not just celebrities. From 1992 to 2003, the number of Americans who admitted to using prescription drugs for nonmedical reasons almost doubled, from 7.8 million to 15.1 million, and abuse among teens more than tripled. Unintentional poisoning deaths—95 percent of which are drug overdoses—increased from 12,186 in 1999 to 20,950 in 2004, according to the CDC. During that time, prescription painkillers, sedatives, and stimulants overtook cocaine and heroin combined as the leading causes of drug fatalities.

The most commonly abused prescription drugs I see include methadone, a drug used to treat heroin addiction and chronic pain; oxycodone, a painkiller that is the active ingredient in OxyContin; benzodiazepines for treating anxiety; hydrocodone, a painkiller; and fentanyl, a powerful painkiller that is generally used to treat cancer patients. Fentanyl can be injected, ingested through lozenges, or administered through skin patches. Misused, it is dangerous. It has a "low therapeutic window," meaning there's not much difference between the amount it takes to treat you and the amount that constitutes an overdose.

I once autopsied a young man—a partial quadriplegic—who had just switched to fentanyl skin patches from an oral painkiller. He was impatient with how slowly the patch took effect. Frustrated, he slapped on more patches than were prescribed. Too much of this highly potent drug seeped into his system, shutting down his central nervous system, and he died in his sleep.

Among the most disturbing aspects of prescription drug abuse is the common misperception that because these medications are prescribed by physicians, they are safe even when used illicitly. Additionally, prescription drugs are often far easier to obtain than street drugs. Some people take advantage of the fact that neither doctors nor consumers tend to think of prescription medications as drugs of abuse. Some come by their pills legitimately but trade them for others, like painkillers, that hold greater appeal because of their more potent high. Some develop a network of doctors, all unknown to one another, from whom they get their prescriptions. Others order their drugs from shady Internet pharmacies.

Stiff Cocktails

Such was the case of a forty-five-year-old mother, Ann Barrett, who was found dead on the floor of a friend's house. Among the clues to her death found by law enforcement was a purse next to her body containing two bottles of recently filled prescription medications. One was the potent and highly addictive pain reliever oxycodone (OxyContin), the other a muscle relaxant, carisoprodol (Soma). What troubled the police was that there were 104 pills missing from the bottles. They weren't sure whether they had a suicide or an accidental overdose on their hands. That's when they called my office.

My investigator went to the scene and reviewed all the circumstances, just like we do on every case. The information he gave me suggested that it was drug related. Ann was a known drug abuser of both heroin and cocaine in the past, but she seemed to have switched to prescription drugs.

Ann lived in Orlando, Florida, with her mother, Sonia, and her teenage daughter, Nessa. Her life had been fraught with hardship, drug abuse, arrests, and suicide attempts. But Ann had not fueled her addiction with drugs scored on the street; she had found a new way to get high—by purchasing prescription narcotics on the Internet, about every two to three weeks, according to her mother.

One fatal mistake that leads to a prescription drug addiction is taking more of the drug than you're prescribed. This misuse creeps into dependence. Your body craves the medication, and you believe that you can't live without it. I suspect this is what happened to Ann.

For years, Ann's mother and daughter tried to reverse her steady slide into addiction. But on one particular evening, her daughter had finally reached the end of her rope. Ann was sitting at the kitchen table, eyes glassy and speech slurred, when Nessa got into an argument with her over her drug abuse. But Ann wasn't interested in hearing a lecture. She got mad, packed some clothes, and stormed off to her girlfriend's house. Ann would never return home to her daughter again. Six days later, an urgent call was made to 911. Emergency medical services and police arrived, but when they got to the victim, Ann was no longer in need of help. She was dead.

While I suspected that prescription drugs had killed Ann, I was less certain as to whether her death was an accident or a suicide. I kept my mind open, because I know there are different ways to interpret information. Some people might look at her and say, "Oh, just another druggie, just another person who abuses drugs," but to me, she was somebody's mother and somebody's daughter, and I wanted to know why she died.

Even though I suspected Ann's death was drug related, as I examined her body externally, I looked very carefully for any indications of foul play or injury. I didn't find much, except one little hint about her life. She had scars from cut marks on her wrist, so it was true that she had tried to commit suicide in the past. To me, it was looking more and more like a suicide, though not to Ann's mother, Sonia, who thought it was an accidental overdose because she had seen it coming.

Only a full autopsy would tell for sure.

After we took identification pictures, it was time to open her up and draw toxicology samples. As with most drug-related cases, I knew that toxicology would be key. Lab tests on fluid samples can check for the presence of thousands of compounds, but the two I was most interested in were those found in Ann's purse, oxycodone and carisoprodol. Both drugs can suppress your brain activity. At levels high enough, they can cause a coma and make you stop breathing.

With toxicology samples taken, I began the routine of inspecting each of Ann's internal organs, looking for any indication of natural disease or injuries that may have killed her. There wasn't a shred of evidence at autopsy that amounted to anything, but drug overdoses don't always leave an obvious calling card.

One key aspect of a case like this is the stomach contents. If Ann took a high dose of oxycodone, as in a suicide, some of those pills would still be in her stomach. Even if the pills had dissolved, she would die before all of the medication got absorbed.

There was only one problem. When I inspected her stomach contents, there were no pills to be found. She had about 200 cc (about a mugful) of tan material that looked like it once enjoyed life as a ham sandwich. But I didn't find any pills. I wondered, could Ann's death not be drug related? I had been presuming it was drugs, but I've been fooled before. Where the autopsy was inconclusive, the toxicology tests would hopefully fill in the blanks.

Five weeks later, the results arrived at the morgue, but they arrived with a twist. According to lab tests, Ann did not have two prescription drugs in her system, she had four. Apparently, Ann didn't take only the pills that were in her purse (oxycodone and carisoprodol), she also took two other prescription drugs: alprazolam, an antianxiety drug, and hydrocodone, a narcotic painkiller. The combination of multiple drugs ingested to boost their effects in the body is known as a drug cocktail.

All four medications were central nervous system depressants, but which one had killed her? While the levels of all four were high, none was high enough to trigger an overdose.

What killed Ann Barrett was a combination of these drugs—a mixed drug toxicity. In other words, Ann did not die from a drug overdose in the classic sense, but from an interaction of multiple drugs that her body simply couldn't tolerate. Taken individually, each of the drugs affects the brain by altering the production of neurotransmitters, chemical compounds that act as messengers between cells in the central nervous system. But with a combination, the effects of the drugs were significantly amplified, resulting in a drastic alteration of neurotransmitters and, as a result, decreased brain function and central nervous system depression. Her breathing slowed and her heart rate weakened. Ann passed out. Within minutes, her brain ceased to function, and without any signal from the brain to prompt respiration, she stopped breathing. Her heart stopped beating and she died.

But why did Ann take the four drugs? To take her own life? Or was it an accidental overdose?

Sometimes working a drug case is like piecing together a mosaic. You can't tell what the whole picture is with a few pieces of tile. What did the autopsy show? What did the toxicology show? What were the circumstances? You have to put every little piece together.

Given that Ann had a history of getting high, the levels of any single drug in her system weren't at suicide-type levels, and that there were no pills detected in her stomach contents, there was little reason to suspect that she had intended to kill herself. I concluded that Ann's mother was right. Ann did not commit suicide.

In the death of Ann Barrett, there was still one unanswered question: If she did not ingest the 104 missing pills, what happened to them? I got the answer from Ann's mother: Ann was selling them to other users. She'd go on the Internet, order drugs, then sell them.

Some of the reasons for the rise in the number of abuse and death cases like Ann's are accessibility through the Internet, doctors who too readily prescribe these powerful drugs, and people who "doctor shop" to obtain multiple prescriptions.

To me, the abuse of prescription drugs is a public health crisis. As a medical examiner, I care about the public health aspects of my cases. Like all medical examiners, I see patterns, take what's learned about the prevalence of disease and death, then examine and determine if there are ways to increase or provide prevention. For example, if I see a lot of deaths due to prescription drug abuse—and I do—then that tells me the community needs to do more to restrict access or educate people about the dangers. What I find on the autopsy table can help society. Laws get changed because of the information medical examiners find out and report, and this helps prevent such heartbreaking deaths as the ones I've described in this chapter.

TURN THE TABLES: Listen to Snoring and Save a Life

Snoring can be more than an annoyance. It can be a sign that someone is slipping into a coma. If a person taking painkillers with or without sedatives begins to snore loudly, but he's not someone who ordinarily snores and you can't rouse him, take it seriously and call 911. That loud snoring might be the relaxing of his pharynx and larynx, signaling that he is about to slip into a coma.

Methamphetamine Madness

Many law-enforcement agents are calling methamphetamine ("meth") abuse the country's most serious—and fastest-growing—drug problem. According to the 2006 National Survey on Drug Use and Health, an estimated 5.77 percent of the U.S. population aged twelve or older have used methamphetamine at least once in their lifetimes. Methamphetamine is a brain-damaging drug. A stimulant similar to cocaine, it causes an intense rush when smoked or injected intravenously and a sense of euphoria when used orally or snorted.

The substance, which can be easily made using household chemicals like lye and cold medicine, has been shown to alter brain cells permanently and cause neurological symptoms similar to those seen in Parkinson's disease. In the short term, methamphetamine use imparts feelings of control and high energy; however, it's so highly addictive that pretty soon, the drug is controlling you.

Methamphetamine causes users to stay up for days at a time without sleeping. I once autopsied a mechanic who was a known abuser. One morning, he got in his old, defective van to go to work after being awake for six days. High on meth, he turned on the ignition and immediately fell asleep. He died of carbon monoxide poisoning and was found badly decomposed three days later.

Methamphetamine itself has a decomposing effect on the body while you're living. It is notorious for ruining a user's appearance—and quickly. Many addicts have black, rotting teeth, worn down to stumps. They tend to scratch nervously (because of a sensation of imaginary bugs crawling under their skin), causing sores and lesions on their bodies. Within a year or two, people seem to age ten years or more. It's not pretty.

One Drug That Probably Won't Kill You

It's been called the demon weed, but marijuana, the most commonly used illegal drug in the United States, has turned out to be less devilish than originally thought. The main active chemical in marijuana is tetrahydrocannabinol (THC). Its short-term effects on the body include memory and learning problems, distorted perception, difficulty thinking and solving problems, and sometimes psychosis—most of which fade if the user stops. I usually don't see it associated with homicides (except those associated with drug deals gone bad), and rarely do I see it associated with driving accidents.

Once during my fellowship in Miami, I autopsied a construction worker who had been working at a site in a ritzy part of town where some exclusive condos were going up. One of the huge booms, used to elevate material, started to tip. Everyone scrambled to get out of the way, except one guy, who just gazed up at it as it came crashing down. It fell on him and cracked his safety helmet and skull wide open.

At first, I didn't think much of it. It was a work-related accident. But then the case started gnawing at me: Why didn't he get out of the way? I carefully examined his trousers, and there I discovered relatively large burn holes. Cigarette ashes wouldn't burn holes that big. Then it hit me: Smoldering seeds that had popped from a marijuana joint could sear large holes in clothes. So I had his blood tested for marijuana, and sure enough, he was very high, even though it was only ten o'clock in the morning. Marijuana can slow down your response time and distort your perception, and that's what happened to him.

In terms of damage to the body, one joint causes a similar degree of lung damage as five cigarettes, and may cause asthma or chronic bronchitis. The jury is still out on whether repeated chestfuls of marijuana smoke increase the risk of cancers of the mouth, throat, and lungs. There's some evidence, however, that smoking weed may promote precancerous changes in the lungs. What's more, recent research suggests that marijuana may increase the risk of psychosis later in life. Reasons enough to stay away from it, if you ask me.

> **LIFE LESSONS: The World's Most Popular Mood-Altering Drug**
>
> Present in coffee, tea, soft drinks, energy drinks, and over-the-counter medicines, caffeine can lift your mood, improve concentration, and boost physical stamina. If you try to abstain from caffeinated beverages, you might suffer withdrawal symptoms such as splitting headaches, nausea, drowsiness, depression, or reduced attention span. By most accounts, though, this stimulant is fairly safe, and there's nothing inherently wrong with being dependent on it. For those accustomed to caffeine, a moderate intake is 200 to 300 milligrams a day—the equivalent of two to three cups of brewed coffee. If you exceed 500 to 600 milligrams, anxiety, nausea, and heart palpitations may set in.

How to Not to Die from Drugs

My patients are dead, so obviously I'm not going to be able to help them get into drug treatment programs. But to those of you who are alive, I have this to say: I don't want you to kill yourself, and if you're doing drugs, you seem to be really trying to—and you need to get help.

Since I don't treat the living, I learn about drug treatment by reading medical literature and talking with my doctor colleagues, including my husband, Dr. Mark Wallace. He's a great resource for me. Often, when we spend some precious moments alone, we discuss medicine, and he keeps me up-to-date on treatments, including drug addiction treatment. Of course, the best way to beat drugs is not to use them in the first place. It's a message you want to share with your kids, too, again and again and again. Mark and I tell our boys rather bluntly that drugs are a road to nowhere.

Addictions are complex. They involve your health, behavior, family life, and work—which is why becoming addiction free is not an easy or quick process. The common starting point, though, is with your doctor, who can get you into the right program.

Usually, the first stage of addiction treatment is medical detoxification, a process whereby you're safely and systemically withdrawn from the addictive drug under medical supervision. Detoxification also helps manage physical withdrawal symptoms. Once you start feeling better, you can move on to more comprehensive rehabilitation.

Rehabilitation helps you address the many health and social problems associated with drug abuse. Depending on the seriousness of your problem, you'll do rehab in a residential program (usually reserved for those whose addiction is so out of control that they can't get well at home), or in an outpatient setting.

Rehab might include, ironically, taking a prescribed drug. Methadone, for example, can be helpful for people addicted to heroin or other opiates, like painkillers. Other useful drugs are naltrexone (Revia) and buprenorphine

(Suboxone). These drugs don't cure addictions. They help people reduce their drug use and pull their lives together while undergoing treatment.

Medications work best when combined with a counseling program. Counseling helps you develop coping skills so you can avoid relapse and improve the likelihood of your long-term treatment success. Many people supplement their counseling with support group meetings, which provide encouragement in less-formal surroundings.

Once you're out of rehab, continuing care is necessary. This involves additional individual, group, and family therapy sessions. It's something you might want to stay with indefinitely to self-manage temptation, cravings, and relapses, and just as important, to help you develop an enjoyable, productive life. See "Resources and Websites" for additional information on getting help for addictions.

If you or someone you know is involved with drugs, it's important to seek treatment as soon as possible, before it's too late. Help is out there.

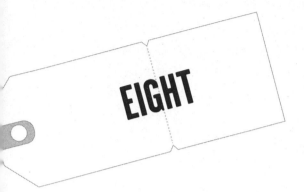

EIGHT

Up in Smoke:
Risking Life and Lung

Mysterious Remains

Sometimes you hook enough red herrings in a death investigation to stock a fish market, and the case of the John Doe lying in my morgue one January morning was one such catch. The night before, two police officers were patrolling one of the roughest neighborhoods in Orlando when the unmistakable sound of gunfire exploded through the air. Moments later came a 911 call. A body had been found just a few blocks from the officers' patrol car.

When the officers arrived on the scene, they were confronted with a strange and horrific sight: The nude body of a man lying facedown in a pool of blood. They suspected he had been shot.

I'm often asked why unidentified bodies are called "John Does." Although its origins are murky, the term probably originated in England under a Magna Carta law stipulating that two witnesses were needed for legal action. To protect their identities, substitute names were often placed on documents. Two of the most-often-used names were John Doe and Richard Roe, perhaps because venison and fish were favorite English foods. A doe is a female deer; roe, a less-familiar term for deer, is also a name for fish eggs. I didn't know much about this John Doe, but as a possible homicide, he would get high priority.

John Doe's face was covered with blood, as was his full head of hair, hinting that he might have been shot, as the police hypothesized. Anytime a gunshot wound is suspected, I first x-ray the body to look for a bullet or for evidence that a bullet had exited, and that's what we did with John Doe. Any bullet or fragments left behind would appear as a white area on the X-ray. When x-raying a body in the morgue, we don't have to worry about overexposure. You can't hurt a dead body with too much radiation.

While I waited on the X-rays, a quick glance at his body revealed a life that was anything but easy. His beard and fingers were stained yellow, and there were deep furrows in his face. His skin was gray, his teeth yellow, and the first two fingers on his right hand jaundiced from the rub of cigarette filters—characteristics I see in heavy smokers. John Doe was clearly among the nearly forty-four million people in the United States who smoke cigarettes—the most lethal habit in the world, one that reduces life expectancy by approximately fourteen years, says the CDC.

Next, my morgue technician wheeled the body out of the X-ray room. Gently and with respect, he bathed and prepped the body. John Doe appeared to be deep in thought: His eyes, slightly open, gazed dreamily at the ceiling.

As soon as the X-rays were ready, I examined the film for bullet fragments and fractures. But there was something strange. After a thorough going-over, I didn't find a bullet, fragments, or trauma. But sometimes trauma from small-caliber gunshot wounds don't show up on X-rays. Also, bullets sometime exit the body, and small-caliber gunshot wounds to the head can be missed on the external examination on someone with a lot of hair.

The only way to know for sure was to open up the man's skull, which we did. I stepped in to do the internal examination of the head. But after a painstaking examination of the inside of the skull cavity, there was still no evidence whatsoever of a head wound. I was sure that this man didn't die from a gunshot wound.

Of course, the case was far from over, and the questions outnumbered the answers. What left him covered in his own blood? And why was he found naked in a parking lot? What killed him? I was back at square one.

As the autopsy posed more questions, the investigation outside the morgue found more answers. John Doe now had a real name.

He was Charles Simmons, a drifter who lived in a vacant, ramshackle apartment. Inside his residence, the police found an important clue for me: tissues soaked with blood.

I went back to his X-rays, hunting for any condition that would cause him to cough up blood. I noticed round whitish areas on his lungs. They appeared to be granulomas, sometimes formed when immune cells surround and engulf bacteria—and a possible sign of tuberculosis. TB is a dangerous infection of the respiratory system that usually occurs when a certain type of bacteria is inhaled into the lungs. Left untreated, TB bacteria will develop these granulomas, which grow in the oxygen-rich air sacs of the lungs. They destroy tissue as they expand, doing enough damage to rupture blood vessels. A person with TB can cough up a tremendous amount of blood.

Not too many pathogens survive after you're dead. TB is different. It remains highly contagious, if not deadly, even after the carrier has died, and contact with a TB victim comes with serious risk. Under ordinary circumstances, we go through huge numbers of disposable gloves, shoe covers, aprons, and other protective clothing. With this case, we also had to wear special masks during the autopsy to protect ourselves against possible infection.

I opened up his chest using the Y incision and inspected his internal organs. His lungs were ravaged with lesions. As I palpated them, the outside surface felt firm where there should be air. The granulomas were calcified, meaning that they contained calcium deposits. Since it takes time for calcium to be deposited in a granuloma, these were probably old ones—an indication that he had contracted TB years before, but it was now dormant. I was convinced that he had at least once suffered from TB. Like the possible gunshot wound, the TB was a red herring, a latent illness that no longer posed a health risk. But this was only the tip of the iceberg. Charles Simmons had a large whitish mass in the top portion of his right lung that had spread deep into the lung tissue and else-where, and I suspected it was cancer.

My suspicions were confirmed once I dissected the mass. It was an advanced case of lung cancer, made even worse by its location and direction of growth.

With this discovery, I was able to piece together the last moments of his life. On the night of his death, Charles Simmons began a violent fit of coughing. Inside his chest, the tumor had dealt its final blow, pushing through the wall of his lung into his pulmonary artery. Like a bursting dam, blood began to flow through the hole, filling his lungs. Unable to cry for help, he probably realized the severity of his condition. I'm sure he panicked—this would be a very scary way to die—and with no time to dress, he hurried out of his apartment and stumbled into the street.

But it was too late. He had lost pints of blood and there was not enough to carry oxygen to his brain. He bled to death from the inside. Somewhere, nearby, a gun was fired—a totally unrelated incident! In the final analysis, it wasn't random urban violence that killed this man, but an unchecked cancer that had been eating through his lungs for years. Incredibly, the man who came into my morgue as a homicide victim left as a victim of disease—a disease brought on undoubtedly by his years of smoking.

As I thought about Charles Simmons, I knew that this was a man who didn't take care of himself, and I often see horrific illnesses like this in people who are transient. There was nobody to look after him, either, so in solving this compli-cated case, perhaps I did something for him in death that others couldn't do for him while he was alive. I cared about him, worked hard to figure out why he had died, and gave him the best that I could.

I can't tell you how to live, but if you're going to smoke or use tobacco—and you don't quit—I can certainly predict that there's a good chance you'll die pre-maturely. Cigarette smoking is the single most preventable cause of premature death and illness worldwide. The reason it's so deadly is that tobacco smoke contains some four thousand compounds, including tar, ammonia, arsenic, cyanide, and carbon monoxide (similar to car exhaust), but it's nicotine, tobacco's most active ingredient, that hooks the user.

When you puff on a cigarette, the smoke and the toxic substances it contains go into your body and some never leave. Eventually, this foreign material is picked up by bloblike cells called macrophages that act like trash collectors in the body. They gather up the debris and landfill it somewhere in the body. For smoke and its constituent toxic garbage, that landfill is the lungs.

I can tell if a dead person was a smoker the minute I see the lungs. Where healthy lungs are pinkish, a smoker's lungs are gray and ribboned with black pigment. When someone has emphysema, which is usually caused by years of smoking, there's a lot of trapped air in the lungs because air isn't exchanged well. A normal lung will keep its shape as you cut it, but emphysema lungs are overinflated. Because of the large amount of trapped air, the rib cage is expanded and the chest is barrel shaped. At autopsy, as soon as I make a cut, the lungs deflate, literally, like you're bursting a balloon but without the pop.

But to return to the addictive nature of nicotine: Not long after taking up the habit, smokers become used to nicotine's effects; as with heroin and cocaine, dependence quickly follows. But unlike those two drugs, nicotine is not likely to fatally overstimulate a healthy heart, cause seizures or coma, or pack anywhere near the same euphoric punch. People who do cocaine can die immediately. With cigarettes, the problems catch up with you later. Nobody lights up their first cigarette and dies. (There's one exception, however: a rare lung disease called eosinophilic pneumonia, which can be fatal in new smokers.) But like cocaine, nicotine causes constriction of the blood vessels and damage to the lining of the arteries with premature buildup of atherosclerotic plaque.

Nicotine stimulates and relaxes the body at the same time. Because it's inhaled, it takes only ten to fifteen seconds after a puff to reach the brain—much faster than intravenous drugs or alcohol. Once there, nicotine attaches to brain cells in a way that causes them to release a flood of neurotransmitters. This action, among other things, affects the reward center of the brain, which encourages people to repeat whatever behavior stimulated it. After a few more puffs, the level of nicotine in the blood soars, the heart beats faster, and blood pressure increases. As a result, smokers become more alert and may actually even think faster. Simultaneously, nicotine may calm the body by churning out natural opiates called endorphins. Thus, if you're a smoker, you can feel alert and relaxed at the same time.

LIFE LESSONS: A Stogie Can Contain as Much Tobacco as a Pack of Cigarettes

Cigars contain the same addictive, toxic, and carcinogenic compounds found in cigarettes and are not a safe alternative to cigarettes. Cigar smokers experience higher rates of lung cancer, heart disease, and chronic obstructive lung disease than nonsmokers. Studies show that men who smoke at least three cigars a day are two to three times more likely to die of lung cancer than nonsmokers. In addition, cigar smoking has similar consequences to cigarette smoking, including four to ten times the risk of dying from oral, esophageal, or laryngeal cancer in comparison to nonsmokers.

Source: Reprinted with permission © 2008 American Lung Association

---

Up in Smoke—and Flames

Nicotine is so addictive that for some smokers, it becomes nearly impossible to give up. In 2007 in my jurisdiction, the Florida Department of Children and Families began investigating David Johnson. He was the forty-two-year-old son of Sara Johnson, who was a constant and careless smoker with a pack-a-day habit. Not surprisingly, Sara, age seventy-six, had emphysema. She had to have oxygen twenty-four hours a day through a mask worn over her face.

David lived with Sara because she required around-the-clock care. Although on oxygen, which is highly flammable, she refused to give up her cigarettes and was constantly trying to smoke under her oxygen mask, often while in bed. Several times in the past Sara had set herself and her house on fire and had to have operations and skin grafts because of it. The reason for the investigation was that David seemingly had not taken her cigarettes away from her, and the authorities wanted to know why.

One Wednesday evening, David awoke to noise coming from his mother's room. He got up and dashed in, only to find her standing up with flames shooting out from under her oxygen mask. She stumbled and fell forward, and David ran to the oxygen control device and shut it off. The flame immediately went out. Sara was badly burned on her lips and nose. David called 911, and Sara was transported to a nearby hospital. Expected to be released after a few days, Sara instead took a turn for the worst and died.

Her body was sent to me to be autopsied. The examination revealed first- and second-degree burns on her face, soot in her nasal cavity, burns on her upper left arm and a finger on her right hand, and contusions on her forehead and elbows. I noted scars on her right breast, the right side of her abdomen, and her right leg, each from previous incidents that told the terrible story of smoking cigarettes while using oxygen. I concluded that what had caused her death was end-stage chronic pulmonary lung disease, which destroyed the lungs' ability to move oxygen into the bloodstream and eventually caused respiratory failure. Contributing to the death were the burns on her face. The manner of death was accidental.

Why did David keep letting his mother smoke—the supposed offense for which he was being investigated? I called him to discuss his mother's death, and from our conversation, learned much more about the personality of a smoker left bereft without cigarettes. "You don't know what she's like when she doesn't have cigarettes. You can't live with her!" he told me. "She turns into a witch. If that's the way she wanted to die, that's the way she wanted to die." And sure enough, that's how she died.

The stress that smokers typically experience when not smoking is induced by nicotine withdrawal, prompting them to feel that they cannot cope with life without cigarettes. When nicotine is unavailable, even for only a few hours, there are uncomfortable withdrawal symptoms that can include anxiety, irritability, difficulty concentrating, restlessness, hunger, craving for tobacco, disturbed sleep, and, in some people, depression. No wonder it's such a tough habit to kick.

LIFE LESSONS: Smokeless Tobacco Contains Twenty-Eight Carcinogens

Smokeless tobacco, in the form of chewing tobacco or snuff, carries significant health risks, including oral cancer, and is not a safe substitute for smoking cigarettes. It also contains nicotine and so can still lead to nicotine addiction. In fact, holding one pinch of smokeless tobacco in your mouth for thirty minutes delivers as much nicotine as three to four cigarettes.

Source: Reprinted with permission © 2008 American Lung Association

---

Puffing Your Way to the Grave

My husband, Mark, and I talk shop occasionally. While I was writing this chapter, he told me that a lot of his patients who are smokers come to his office, worried about their cholesterol levels, wanting to have their PSA checked for prostate cancer, or anxious about eating pesticides in food. These concerns are all valid, but Mark's patients blithely ignore the major thing that really will send them to an early grave: smoking.

Smoking is the most destructive thing you can do to your body and claims an estimated 430,700 American lives each year, according to the American Lung Association. It's responsible for about 30 percent of cancer deaths, 87 percent of lung cancer cases, and 20 percent of cardiovascular deaths in the United States. Further, it causes most cases of emphysema and chronic bronchitis. Cigarette smoking also weakens your bones, particularly in the hip, leading to osteoporosis. In the elderly, there's a high mortality rate associated with hip fractures.

DEADLY DANGERS OF SMOKING

Cardiovascular disease	Arrhythmia
	Heart attack
	Unstable angina
	Stroke
	Blocked arteries
	Aortic aneurysm
Pulmonary disease	Lung cancer
	Chronic bronchitis
	Emphysema
	Asthma
	Increased susceptibility to pneumonia
	Increased susceptibility to pulmonary tuberculosis
Gastrointestinal	Peptic ulcer
	Gastroesophageal reflux disease (GERD)
	Crohn's disease
Reproductive	Reduced fertility
	Premature birth
	Low birth weight
	Spontaneous abortion
	Prenatal mortality
Oral	Leukoplakia (patchy white spots on the mucous membranes in the mouth)
	Gingivitis
	Gingival recession
	Tooth staining

Other	Cancers of the larynx, oral cavity, esophagus, pancreas, bladder, kidney, stomach, and cervix, and leukemia
	Type 2 diabetes
	Erectile dysfunction
	Early menopause
	Osteoporosis
	Cataracts
	Age-related macular degeneration
	Premature skin wrinkling
	Graves' disease
	Aggravation of hypothyroidism
	Interactions with prescription drugs

By His Own Hand

Recently, I autopsied a fifty-three-year-old smoker, Rob Allen, who was plagued by a number of these smoking-related problems, including chronic lung disease and coronary artery disease. He had once been treated for lung cancer, as well as for head and neck malignancies. Rob had to have a hole surgically cut in his neck and a breathing tube inserted so he could breathe. Nevertheless, he continued to smoke and did so through the breathing tube. A few years later, it was found that the lung cancer had reappeared, and Rob was terminally ill. After being told the news by his doctor, Rob took a spin in his sports car, parked it, and smoked a cigarette.

Many hours later, he was reported missing, and deputies began a search. They found Rob and his car on a lonely stretch of road. He had put a gun to his head and killed himself—a self-inflicted death that would later be confirmed in my autopsy. How do I know he had one last smoke? Found next to his body were his cigarettes and lighter. For Rob, life had become a bitter and unbearable burden, and he had decided it wasn't worth living. Technically, that's not a

Protect Yourself and Your Family from Secondhand Smoke

- Never smoke in your home or around children. Many of the toxic substances linger in the air even after the cigarette, cigar, or pipe is gone.
- Ask other people not to smoke in your home, especially babysitters, relatives, and others who care for your children.
- Make certain that your children's day-care centers, schools, restaurants, and other places your family spends time in are smoke free.
- Be assertive: Let family, friends, and the people you work with know that you *do* care if they smoke around you.
- In restaurants and bars, ask to sit in the nonsmoking area.
- Ask your employer to make sure you do not have to breathe other people's smoke at work.
- Quit smoking, for yourself and your loved ones.

Source: Reprinted with permission © American Lung Association

death caused by smoking, and I can't put smoking on the death certificate, but I can guarantee it was the true killer.

There are so many medical problems associated with smoking that it's best for me to list them for you in the table on page 169.

Secondhand Smoke SOS

I don't smoke cigarettes—never have and never will—and I've always been careful about another killer: breathing secondhand smoke. The health risks of inhaling a little of the stuff at home, in a bar or restaurant, or at a building entranceway are well documented. Secondhand smoke contains at least 250 chemicals known to be toxic, including more than 50 that can cause cancer. Exposure to secondhand smoke is estimated to cause forty-six thousand heart disease deaths in adult nonsmokers in the United States each year, says the American Lung Association. Based on scientific evidence, the most recent Surgeon General's Report has concluded that there is no risk-free level of exposure to secondhand smoke. Even brief exposures to secondhand smoke can damage the lining of blood vessels, decrease coronary blood flow, and compromise your heart rate, potentially increasing the risk of heart attack. The damage isn't just to your ticker, either. Breathing in secondhand smoke causes approximately 3,400 lung cancer deaths annually.

If you smoke, kick the habit for your kids' health. Secondhand smoke is highly dangerous for children. Your kids will have a greater chance of developing asthma, ear infections, bronchitis, pneumonia, sinusitis, allergies, and pulmonary infections. Also linked to secondhand smoke is sudden infant death syndrome (SIDS), something I sadly see in the morgue all too frequently.

How Not to Die from Smoking

There's a far more important fact than these ominous statistics and tragic stories, and it is this: Smokers can quit and there are more ways to do so than ever. Although it is not easy, countless millions have quit, and you can, too. Your first step should be to see your doctor to discuss smoking-cessation therapies. There's a whole pack of treatments and therapies that can take some of the pain out of quitting. Here are some of the most effective techniques.

Nicotine-Replacement Therapy

Nicotine-replacement therapy is designed to lessen the acute symptoms of withdrawal, such as irritability, sleeplessness, and anxiety. It also helps control cravings as you wean yourself off nicotine. Nowadays you have a choice among gum, lozenges, skin patches, inhalers, or nasal sprays. These substitutes still deliver nicotine to your bloodstream, but more slowly than smoking and at a lower dose. Although recommended by the manufacturer for relatively short-term use (generally three to six months), the use of these methods for six months or longer is safe and may be helpful if you're afraid of relapsing without them. Patches, which slowly release nicotine through the skin, are a good choice if you suffer from nasal allergies or sinusitis. Pregnant women, heart patients, and folks with high blood pressure should not use nicotine substitutes except under a doctor's supervision.

Antismoking Pills

Currently, two medications (besides nicotine) are approved for smoking cessation: bupropion and varenicline. Bupropion, sold under the brand name Zyban, is a prescription drug that works on the brain to lessen the symptoms of nicotine withdrawal. It has also been used under the name Wellbutrin to treat people for depression. People who take Zyban tend not to gain weight when they quit smoking, which is one of its advantages. The drug can be used alone or, to increase your chances of success, in combination with a nicotine patch. Zyban is not for you, however, if you suffer a seizure disorder, have ever had a head injury or stroke, or already take Wellbutrin or certain other antidepressants.

Varenicline (Chantix) helps you quit smoking by blocking nicotine receptors in the brain and killing your cravings for nicotine. You begin taking the drug seven days before you stop smoking and continue taking it for twelve weeks or longer. It often requires several attempts to successfully quit smoking. Should a relapse occur, your doctor will probably advise you to keep taking the drug and try again. The Chantix label warns doctors to monitor their patients for

> **TURN THE TABLES: Smoking Stoppers**
> Try to get oral gratification in other ways. Suck on sugar-free mints. Chew sugar-free gum. Cut a straw up into the size of a cigarette and keep it in your mouth. Or sip herbal tea. These substitutions may take away your desire to smoke.

neuropsychiatric symptoms, such as changes in behavior, agitation, depressed mood, suicidal thoughts, and suicidal behavior. If you've had any sort of pre-existing psychiatric illness, it's probably not a good idea to take this drug as it may aggravate mood swings.

Start Sweating, Stop Smoking

A regular exercise program can be a quitter's best friend. Researchers at Brown University found that quitters who worked out were twice as likely to stay cigarette free for at least one year after quitting as those who didn't exercise. The suspected reason? Spiked endorphin levels help counteract the symptoms of nicotine withdrawal. Exercise also helped prevent weight gain (typical in people who quit smoking), probably by giving a boost to the metabolism. Many other studies have demonstrated that exercise should be a part of a treatment program for nicotine dependence.

HOW YOUR BODY CHANGES AFTER YOU QUIT SMOKING

20 minutes after you quit:

• Your blood pressure decreases.

• Your pulse rate drops.

• The temperature of your hands and feet increases.

8 hours after you quit:

• The carbon monoxide level in your blood drops to normal.

• The oxygen level in your blood increases to normal.

24 hours after you quit.

• Your likelihood of having a heart attack decreases.

48 hours after you quit:

• Your nerve endings start regrowing.

• Your taste buds and ability to smell improve.

2 to 3 months after you quit:

• Your circulation improves.

• Walking becomes easier.

• Your lung function increases.

Up to 9 months after you quit:

• You'll have less coughing, sinus congestion, and shortness of breath.

• You'll have more energy.

1 year after you quit:

• Your risk of coronary heart disease decreases to half that of a smoker.

5 years after you quit:

• From 5 to 15 years after quitting, your stroke risk is reduced to that of people who have never smoked.

10 years after you quit:

• Your risk of lung cancer drops to as little as one-half that of continuing smokers.

• Your risk of cancers of the mouth, throat, esophagus, bladder, kidney, and pancreas decreases.

• Your risk of ulcer decreases.

15 years after you quit:

• Your risk of coronary heart disease is now similar to that of people who have never smoked.

• Your risk of death returns to nearly the level of people who have never smoked.

Source: Reprinted with permission © 2008 American Lung Association

Other Ways to Quit This Bad Habit

Whatever method you and your doctor decide to use, two other keys to success may help: good social support from family and friends or a self-help group like Nicotine Anonymous, and a program that offers "skills training." These groups show you how to cope with cravings and high-risk situations that trigger a desire to smoke, as well as teach stress management and relaxation techniques. You'll also learn how to start changing your smoking patterns. That way, the associations (like having a cigarette with coffee or an alcoholic beverage), are disrupted, and you're less likely to mindlessly reach for a cigarette. Also, if you smoke, I urge you to get all the information you can about quitting from groups like the American Cancer Society, the American Heart Association, and the American Lung Association. Finally, it may take several attempts before you actually quit. If one method doesn't work, try the next and the next, until you ultimately hit on something that does.

The Benefits of Being a Quitter

It's never too late to quit, but the sooner you do, the better. As the smoke-free years go by, your risk of heart disease, stroke, and lung disease diminish until they are essentially the same as that of a person who has never smoked. Someone who quits smoking at the age of fifty-five, for example, has half the risk of dying of lung cancer compared with a continuing smoker. The risk of a heart attack falls rapidly after quitting smoking and approaches nonsmoking levels within a few years of being smoke free. No matter how long you've been smoking, your body can repair much of the damage that has been done by smoking. After you quit, your body will begin to function more efficiently. You'll feel better and look better, and be healthier to boot.

Best of all, a smoke-free life will help keep you from seeing me for many years to come.

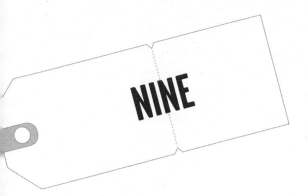

NINE

Everyday Dangers

Falling Down Dead

During the winter of 2003, a brutal ice storm swept into Kirby, Texas, while I was serving as the medical examiner at the Bexar County Morgue. Temperatures dropped to below twenty degrees—that's unusual for Texas—and everything was frozen over.

There were several deaths in the storm's wake, and one of them was that of ninety-two-year-old Richard Adler, a widower, who was discovered dead in his yard the morning after the storm. Stubbornly independent, he lived alone with the help of a caregiver, despite his age and a diagnosis of dementia. He tried to take care of himself as best he could, which was why the circumstances of his death were so disturbing.

According to Richard's caregiver, Mary, she arrived at his house at 9 a.m. as usual, only to find his front door wide open and no signs of him inside the cold house. Worried, she searched all over the house but could not find him. Approaching the backyard, Mary noticed that the fence gate was ajar. Then she saw him—facedown on the frozen ground by the raised cement patio. There were cuts and bruises all over his body, and he was clearly no longer alive. In addition, the screen door was covered with blood. His glasses were bloody, too. My investigator and the police were dispatched to the scene.

They suspected that perhaps he had been the victim of a home-invasion robbery. Although robberies have decreased overall in the United States, at the time of Richard's death, home invasions, which typically target the elderly, were on the rise.

In addition, he might have fallen off the cement patio—a fall that could have killed him. My investigator found marks on the ground near Richard's feet, suggesting that he had been moving a little bit and pushing the dirt around after the fall. He also showed signs of a struggle, as though he had been grabbing at something in the mud.

The authorities contacted his family, and they were understandably distraught, particularly over what he may have endured during his final hours. How long was he there? Did he suffer? Or did he die right away?

Like any unexplained fatality, the death of Richard Adler would require a full autopsy.

As part of the external examination, I collected forensic evidence from his fingernails in the event that he had been attacked. So that I could get a better look at his injuries, my morgue technician stripped his body and washed it of debris. Once the body was cleaned, the trauma was evident. I noted that there were bruises and abrasions on his elbows, a bruise on the back of his left hand, and a deep tear that exposed the ligaments in his hand. The severity of the trauma added to the burning question: What did this man endure before he died?

Before completing the external examination, I checked to see if Richard had broken a hip. If so, he joined a group of more than 350,000 elderly Americans who fracture their hips each year. At ninety-two and suffering from dementia, Richard was in one of the highest-risk groups for this type of accident. The incidence of hip fractures not only increases after age fifty but doubles every five to six years as the risk of falling increases. Slipping and tumbling are not the only causes of hip fractures; weakened bones sometimes break with minimal trauma. But falling is the major cause, representing 90 percent of all hip fractures. These injuries are not to be taken lightly. According to the American Academy of Orthopaedic Surgeons, only 25 percent of those who suffer hip fractures ever fully recover; as many as 20 percent will die within twelve months. Even when patients do recover, nearly half need a cane or a walker to get around.

If Richard had broken a hip, it would be one reason why he had been lying there, unable to get up. But I found no indication of a fracture.

I opened his frail, thin body with the Y incision. What was immediately clear was Richard's poor state of health. His lungs showed signs of emphysema. His heart was weakened from years of plaque buildup in his coronary arteries. It was enlarged and heavy, too, as if he was chronically hypertensive, and was dilating, meaning that it had started to fail.

After removing every organ from his body, I inspected the inside of his abdominal cavity for any internal injuries—and I found something unusual. Richard Adler had six broken ribs along his back—clear signs of trauma.

The six ribs were broken in a clear distinct line that stretched to the spine, which was also broken. By far the most likely way for an injury like this to occur is an impact against a hard edge (like the lip of a cement patio) and not from a blow from a fist. In a young person, a fall like that might result in a minor injury, but in a ninety-two-year-old, such a fall would be devastating.

I now believed that trauma was involved in Richard's death, but I also concluded that his heart and lungs were contributing factors. Fractured bones place a lot of stress on your body and can cause pain. Add to these factors the cold weather, and a diseased heart cannot keep pace.

But if Richard had died from the fall, this would explain only one part of the troubling death scene. Still unknown was what he was doing in the backyard in the first place—and why he fell. I hoped that the clues to help me understand this complex case could be found in his brain.

My morgue technician opened his skull. First, I inspected the top of the skull to make sure he didn't suffer a blow to the head. I didn't find anything abnormal such as a contusion or bruise after reflecting, or peeling back, his scalp.

Then I examined the brain itself, and there I did find an abnormality, but it was not trauma. It was brain atrophy. Mr. Adler's brain had shrunk, and there were wide-open gaps between the gyri, the coral-like folds of the brain. The loss of tissue in his brain was typical of what you'd see in advanced-stage dementia.

Dementia is a disorder caused by the death or impairment of nerve cells in the brain. There are many kinds of dementia, but the most common in people sixty-five and older is Alzheimer's disease, which typically causes memory loss, confusion, agitation, and depression. For me the forensic evidence of dementia, which was confirmed microscopically in Richard's brain, was crucial, and from it, I was able to surmise what had led to his death.

Based on my investigator's report, I knew that Richard's caregiver had left his home at approximately 2:30 p.m. as she usually did. Sometime in the late afternoon, Richard was drawn outside, though not to confront an intruder. He most likely went out to check his mail and left the door ajar. Despite the cold weather, he did not wear a jacket.

But the day's mail had not yet arrived. Perhaps at that moment, the elderly man, suffering from advanced dementia, suddenly became confused. Rather than return inside through the wide-open front door, he walked around to the back door. It was locked, and Richard, already confused, may have become agitated. He probably panicked, trying to get inside, and he cut his knuckles on the torn screen. He tried to take his glasses off because they got covered with blood. Confused, blinded, bleeding across the hands and knuckles, Richard walked across the ice-covered cement patio. With his glasses off, he didn't notice that the surface was slick until it was too late. He fell off the patio, breaking his ribs and spine. The fall exacted a fatal toll. He struggled to breathe. His heart, weakened by disease and the stress of the trauma and cold, fell into a deadly arrhythmia and ceased to beat.

Based on the devastating extent of his injuries and his poor health, I believed that the frail, elderly man likely succumbed quickly. After I talked to his family, they were at least relieved to know that Richard didn't spend the night out in the cold, suffering.

Every five minutes in this country, someone dies from an accident. Accidents encompass a very broad category that includes a lot of stuff that just happens, but in medical examiner lingo, we define "accident" as an unintended, unexpected event resulting in injury or death.

However you define them, accidents are one of the most serious public health issues we face. Across all age groups, they are the fifth leading cause of death. Yet, if you break accident statistics down by age group, you get a completely different picture. For people between the ages of one and forty-four, accidents are the number one killer. That's scary to me. You can eat fiber until it comes out of your ears, then fall off a ladder and die.

Which accidents are the most deadly? Data from the National Safety Council (NSC) shows that poisoning—particularly from overdoses of prescription and illicit drugs—is now the fastest-rising cause of nonvehicular accidental death. Death from a fall ranks second, with choking, drowning, and fires rounding out the top five. These account for 83 percent of all accidental deaths in adults and children.

How Not to Die from Accidents

There are hundreds of accidents that can befall us, and I can't cover them all in one chapter, so I'll talk about accidents that happen to grown-ups and kids in the most dangerous place on earth: your home. Believe it or not, more than fifteen thousand people suffer fatal accidents at home each year in America, and the greatest proportion of those die from falls. In fact, the number of people who suffer fatal falls at home is greater than the number of combined deaths from electrocution, poisoning by gas, lightning, floods, tornadoes, polio, meningitis, and fireworks. Staying less accident-prone may predict whether you make it to old age or not, so I'll give you some guidelines for thinking your way clear of accidents.

Don't Be a Fall Guy or Gal

Falling is a serious problem, particularly for the elderly, as the case of Richard Adler shows. Often, they're shut in their homes, with no one to help them. Another case was that of Jane Mueller, who lived in a Kissimmee apartment. No one had heard from her in a while, so her friends called the police to do a welfare check. Jane was a real clutter bug, with stuff strewn everywhere in her apartment. There was one little path through the clutter, and she was found at the end of the strip, facedown. On closer inspection, investigators found she had been carrying a hairbrush in her hand with the end pointed upward. She tripped and fell on an uneven rug, and the end of the brush went through her eye and into her brain. She died in a puddle of blood from an accidental fall, in a most unusual yet tragic way.

For me, the deaths of Jane Mueller, Richard Adler, and others like them are especially poignant. They show the difficult struggle the elderly face maintaining their independence as they age. It's an issue I have encountered with my own eighty-eight-year-old mother, who like Jane and Richard, lives alone. She's already fallen once, and I'm worried that she'll fall again and no one will be there. But she likes being in her own house, and it's her decision to live alone—a decision she has a right to make, and I have to respect it.

All of us—no matter how old or how young—can take precautions to prevent falls:

- Keep your muscles and bones strong by following an exercise program.
- Don't forget to get sufficient calcium and vitamin D, two critical factors in developing strong bones. These nutrients are available in fortified dairy products.

- Make your home safer with simple improvements, such as good lighting to eliminate dark areas; slip-resistant walking surfaces; grab bars and a night-light in the bathroom; and handrails on stairs.
- Remove throw rugs from doorways and hallways. They often fold over or bunch up, turning them into booby traps for anyone shuffling down the hall.
- Keep your home or apartment free from clutter.
- Practice good ladder safety by having someone hold the ladder while you work.
- Wear shoes with good support, leather soles, and rubber heels.
- Rearrange the furniture throughout your home, so that the paths between rooms are free of obstructions. Also, make sure telephone and appliance cords aren't strung across floors, where they can be tripped over.
- If you have fallen before, consider a full physical evaluation and balance screening, as well as vision and hearing tests.

Falls, of course, aren't the only household accident that can happen. There are other things in your home that can seem like they're out to get you. The checklist on page 184 can help you identify—and eliminate—everyday dangers in your house.

Monoxide Menace

The Senseless Killer

The morgue team stood waiting for me in the autopsy suite one May morning in 2005. There were six bodies lying there—three adults, two teenage boys, and one seven-year-old boy, all related to one another. Their bodies had turned cherry red, the classic sign of carbon monoxide poisoning. As I entered the room, everyone was speculating about whether this could be a mass murder or a murder-suicide.

ACCIDENT-PROOF YOUR HOME: A CHECKLIST

Living Room

Are lamp, extension, and phone cords out of the way of foot traffic?

Are passageways free of clutter?

Do small rugs and runners stay put?

Are curtains and furniture at least twelve inches from baseboard heaters?

Does your fireplace have a good screen to catch sparks?

Has your chimney been inspected and cleaned during the past year?

Has your furnace been serviced professionally in the past year?

Kitchen

Do you keep paper towels, hand towels, curtains, and other things that can burn away from the burners and oven?

Are stove tops and counters clean and free of grease?

Do you turn pot handles inward so that they can't be bumped?

Are kitchen appliances, such as your coffeemaker, toaster, and microwave, plugged into separate receptacle outlets?

Bedrooms

Do you have a carbon monoxide detector near each occupied bedroom?

Is your phone within easy reach of your bed?

Do you have a light or lamp within easy reach of your bed?

Bathrooms

Does your tub or shower have a nonskid surface, such as a mat, decals, or abrasive strips?

Does the tub or shower have a sturdy grab bar?

Do you keep your hot water temperature 120 degrees or lower?

Entrances

Do all entrances have outdoor lights?

Are walkways free from cracks and holes?

Is your address marked outside in large, clear numbers so emergency personnel can find your house quickly?

Throughout Your Home

Have you taken steps to reduce tripping and slipping hazards in your home?

Is there at least one smoke alarm on every floor of your house?

Do you have a fire extinguisher?

Have you developed a fire escape plan?

Do you replace worn or frayed cords promptly, and never run them under furniture or carpeting?

Do you keep emergency phone numbers by the telephone or put them on your speed dial?

Do you keep medicine and household cleaning solutions out of the reach of children?

The victims were residents of a subdivision in Orlando and lived in a neat, orderly three-bedroom home. At around 5:15 p.m. on May 29, a neighbor and close friend, Harold Miller, who had a key to the home, sensed something was wrong. He had not been able to reach anyone at the house for three days and learned that the kids had not gone to school. Worried, Harold decided to check on the family. He smelled car exhaust as soon as he walked into the home. Upon entering the bedrooms, he was horrified to see the bodies lying in natural sleep positions but obviously not alive. He immediately left the home and called the police.

The police and fire department arrived promptly and found the home filled with lethal levels of carbon monoxide. There was no evidence of foul play and no notes were found. A car, a Corolla, had apparently been left running in a closed garage. Once the home was cleared of the gas, my investigators entered the house to begin their investigation. They collected the bodies and claimed them under the jurisdiction of the District Nine Medical Examiner's Office.

As the investigation unfolded, clues to the mystery emerged. Apparently, the uncle had parked his car in the garage and forgot that it was running. The car's exhaust was dangerously close to an intake pipe for the home's air conditioner. Carbon monoxide collected in the garage and then steadily seeped into the house, poisoning the uncle, his niece, her husband, and their three children as they slept. Sadly, I have had several cases like this in which someone accidentally leaves a car running in the garage, killing themselves and other family members. Carbon monoxide poisonings like this can occur even with the garage door left open.

Carbon monoxide has been called "the senseless killer" because it is a colorless, odorless, and tasteless gas and thus nearly impossible for the human senses to detect. When inhaled, it quickly crowds out oxygen molecules that normally attach themselves to the hemoglobin molecules in red blood cells. The carbon monoxide–hemoglobin bond is more than two hundred times stronger than the oxygen-hemoglobin bond. As a result, not enough life-sustaining oxygen gets to tissues, causing illness and sometimes death—as in the case of this family or of suicide victims who run hoses from the engine exhaust to the inside of their cars. Each year, carbon monoxide poisoning contributes to an average of five hundred unintentional deaths and two thousand suicides in the United States, and accounts for roughly fifteen thousand emergency-room visits, according to the CDC.

Carbon monoxide is a by-product of the incomplete combustion of carbon-based fuels such as natural gas, gasoline, kerosene, and wood. Inside your home, fuel-based furnaces, space heaters, water heaters, clothes dryers, and fireplaces typically produce some carbon monoxide. Outside, gasoline-powered engines, such as those in cars, lawn mowers, and generators, emit carbon monoxide as well. When properly ventilated and in good working order, all are safe to use, but potentially deadly problems may arise when they are not. That being so, how can you ensure that your home is safe from carbon monoxide?

- Check for clues that may indicate a problem: excessive condensation on walls and windows; a damaged, rusty, or sooty furnace, heater, chimney, or flue; stale, smelly air (a sign of improper ventilation); or a furnace that runs constantly or fails to heat the house adequately.

- Be aware of physical symptoms, since the human body may also give indications of carbon monoxide buildup in the home. Headache, fatigue, nausea, vomiting, lethargy, and general flu-like symptoms are the most common symptoms of low-level poisoning.

- Have your heating system, water heater, and any other gas-, oil-, or coal-burning appliances serviced by a qualified technician every year. A chimney sweep should clean and inspect your fireplace and chimney, too. Follow the advice of these experts, and have them make the repairs needed to keep your home safe and healthy.

- Invest in carbon monoxide alarms and install them on every floor of your home, especially near sleeping areas.

- Don't use a generator, charcoal grill, camp stove, or other gasoline- or charcoal-burning device inside your home, basement, or garage, or near an open window.

- Don't leave engines running inside your garage or use your oven or stove to heat the house. Never burn charcoal inside your house, even in the fireplace.

⌐ For Kids' Sake

A Freak Accident

Although most of my annual caseload involves adult corpses, many times I must autopsy children. Every case that comes through my morgue is tragic in some way, but the bodies of children who end up here are, without question, the most agonizing of all. They are tragic reminders that even children can't escape untimely and premature deaths. While I was serving as medical examiner in Texas during the 1990s, the police called me one day and announced they were bringing me the body of seventeen-month-old Danny Kansler.

The day before, Charlotte Kansler, Danny's mom, began a morning ritual familiar to most working parents. Before heading off to work, she left young Danny in the hands of a trusted babysitter who cared for several neighborhood children on a regular basis. It was the last time Charlotte would ever see her little boy alive. A few hours later, the police received a panicked 911 call.

Babysitter Hillary Turner claimed to have found Danny in his playpen, unconscious and not breathing. Lifted by helicopter to a local hospital, Danny died en route.

Hillary told the police that Danny's death was a freak accident and that she had found him already unconscious when she checked on him. But when an emergency-room doctor later examined the dead little boy, he made a troubling diagnosis after finding bruising on Danny's neck. The doctor told police Danny had been strangled. They brought in Hillary on suspicion of murder. But for a formal charge to be levied, I had to declare a ruling of homicide.

When the baby's body arrived at my morgue, I could see right away what had alarmed the ER doctor. Along with bruises on the front of his neck, I found two parallel linear abrasions on the top of the head and a linear contusion on the back of his neck. Danny also had small red spots on his face and eyes. These tiny spots, medically called petechiae, can occur because of bleeding under the skin. Often during strangulation, blood continues to pump into the head through the arteries. But the force of the strangulation stops blood from freely flowing back out of the head. Like an overfilled balloon, the resulting pressure ruptures the small vessels, causing the petechiae.

I couldn't really deduce much from this, however. It didn't look like a straightforward strangulation to me. The only thing I knew was that the babysitter found the child unresponsive, and the circumstances were unclear. The investigator's field report didn't describe the nature of the "freak accident" the babysitter claimed had taken place. The case was hazy to me. I didn't want to make any snap judgments, either, since the only thing standing between the babysitter and a murder trial was my ruling. So I made it clear that I wouldn't be rushed.

I do enough autopsies on children who are murdered, unfortunately, to know that people do not usually kill babies by strangling them. This case just wasn't making sense, and there weren't enough findings to put the remaining pieces of the puzzle together. That's when I decided we needed more information to get to the truth.

I called in my field investigators and asked them to return to the crime scene with the police, reenact the baby's death, and photograph that re-creation. Everything had to be carefully documented: the sequence of events, the way the room looked the day of the death, and so forth. Normally, I wouldn't send investigators back to the scene after the body has been removed, but there are times when I can't answer all questions in the autopsy suite. I need additional photographic evidence to see if the story fits the autopsy findings.

Back at the scene, with police and field investigators observing, Hillary told her whole story. The playpen was placed back in the position of the day of the death, and a large doll was used to represent the child.

Hillary explained that Danny Kansler was an overly active toddler who often managed to climb out of his playpen. Hillary, who had other children in her care, told Danny's mother that she needed a way to keep the child from wandering around unsupervised. Together, they came up with a seemingly simple measure to solve the problem. They decided to place something over the top of the playpen so Danny could not get out. What they chose was an empty bed frame on which you'd normally place a mattress, and it had springs strung across it. Hillary added that a plastic tub filled with toys was sitting on an end table near the playpen. She left the room that morning so that Danny could take his nap.

The investigators took photographs of the crib and surrounding area. Then based on Hillary's account, they reconfigured the scene to show how everything looked when she returned. As she entered the room, the tub of toys was on top of the bed frame, and Danny's neck was wedged between the edge of the bed frame and the edge of the playpen. Horrified, Hillary removed Danny immediately and tried to revive him, then called 911.

Back at the morgue, I examined the new photographic evidence and was able to see how the babysitter's explanation matched perfectly with the marks on Danny's neck. The pattern of injury was what I would expect to see if the child was in that position. Everything then came into focus, and I was able to put together the most likely series of events that led to Danny's death.

Originally what was thought to be a strangulation homicide turned out to be an accidental death caused by entrapment and strangulation. With the truth in hand, I called the police and told them to stop their criminal investigation. Hillary Turner was innocent. Danny's mother, Charlotte, though in the grip of grief, told me she was thankful that I had cleared her friend of any wrongdoing.

The world is an exciting place for infants and small children, who love to explore but aren't aware of the potential dangers. Being a parent myself, I know how hard it is to make your home risk free. You really do have to keep an eye on your kids all the time—which is why parents are so exhausted. There are many tragic, senseless accidents involving children every year, and I believe it is crucial to address them here. The ones I see most frequently involve sleeping accidents, choking, animal bites, burns, kids left in unattended vehicles, drowning, and gun accidents.

When Kids Die Before They Wake

Many of the accidental deaths I see in infants are the result of suffocation, and most of these deaths occur because babies are placed in "unsafe sleep environments." What I mean by that is a situation that does not meet guidelines for infant safety and can cause suffocation. Some examples are a child's head or face covered by soft bedding; environments not specifically designed for infants, including adult beds, couches, cushioned chairs, or sleeping with one or more persons; and entrapment in a space through which a portion of the body had passed, such as what happened to little Danny Kansler. You can protect your children from such dangers by making sure that they always sleep in child-appropriate cribs, bassinets, or beds. Be sure to place the crib far away from window treatments and cords. Infants can get tangled in cords and strangle themselves. Always tie up window blind cords so they are out of your child's reach.

Red Alert: Choking Hazards

I see a lot of kids who die from choking on food or objects that easily lodged in their small airways. Anything that fits can be a danger. A few years ago, a seven-month-old baby arrived at the morgue. He had been found dead in his crib, a suspected case of SIDS. Since SIDS usually strikes infants who are two to four

---

Is It SIDS or Is It Unsafe Sleep Practices?

Sudden infant death syndrome, better known as SIDS, is a cruel killer, striking infants as they sleep. It is the third leading cause of infant mortality in the United States, and most SIDS deaths occur between two and four months of age, although the official definition is under one year of age. No one knows for sure what prompts seemingly healthy babies to suddenly die in their sleep, although some experts attribute the sudden deaths to a brain defect, which may impair breathing reflexes, or an electrical defect in the heart.

Today, even when a child seems to die a SIDS death, many medical examiners—myself included—feel compelled to view the case more skeptically. SIDS is a catchall term for unexplained infant deaths and probably has more than one cause.

When you start thoroughly investigating and analyzing some of these cases, you discover a lot of things, such as unsafe sleep practices. Infants are left to sleep on sofas, for instance, or in cribs with toys and bedding that can smother, or in an adult bed, often with multiple people. All of these circumstances may convince me that a death was caused by suffocation (obstruction of the nose and mouth), positional asphyxia (when the body is in a position that it can't breathe), or mechanical asphyxia (crushing). Depending on the case, I might write any of these three on the death certificate when others might have written SIDS.

months old, I was suspicious. I did an autopsy and found a balloon obstructing the child's airway. As it turned out, his older brother had been playing with a balloon. It popped, and he gave it to the baby to play with.

Putting things in their mouths is one of the ways that babies and small children explore the world, so as a parent you have to be eagle-eyed all the time. Teach your kids to chew and swallow their food before talking or laughing. Since kids can choke on any type of food, monitor what they eat and cut foods into small pieces before giving them to your child. Always follow all manufacturers' age recommendations when buying toys. Some toys have small or loose parts that can cause choking, so heed all warnings on a toy's packaging. Teach your children not to put pencils, crayons, or erasers in their mouths when coloring or drawing.

> **TURN THE TABLES: Be Ready in an Emergency**
>
> Post a chart illustrating emergency procedures—such as CPR and the Heimlich maneuver—on your refrigerator.

Dog-Proof Your Kids

Each year, eight hundred thousand Americans seek medical attention for dog bites, and half are children. In fact, the rate of dog-bite-related injuries is highest for kids ages five to nine years old. One of the most horrific cases I ever autopsied was a four-year-old boy who chased his ball into a neighboring yard where four pit pulls were tied up. Although tethered to a post, the dogs were still able to attack him, and the child died of multiple bite wounds. Dog bites are a largely preventable public health problem, and there is a lot you can do to protect yourself and your kids. Get a suitable breed, for example, one that gets along well with kids. Have your dog properly trained to obey basic commands. Socialize your dog so it feels comfortable around people and other animals. Teach your children proper behavior around any dog—yours or someone else's. And never tie or chain your dog up; this tends to make dogs more aggressive.

Is Something Burning?

Burns, especially due to kitchen accidents, are some of the most tragic childhood accidents I see. Babies and children are more susceptible to burns than adults because they have very sensitive skin. I remember a case involving a three-year-old boy who was watching his grandmother cook a big pot of beans on a hot stove. Curious, he reached up and grabbed the pot handle. The whole pot of boiling beans fell on top of him, and he died from the burns. It's just common sense, but keep your kids away from anything that's hot, such as the stove, oven, hot foods or beverages, radiators, and electric baseboard heaters.

Unattended Kids in Cars

At least once a year, I get a case involving a parent who unintentionally left a child in a car, and the child died of heat stroke. Children are especially susceptible to heat stroke because their core body temperatures rise three to five times faster than that of adults. This can occur within minutes.

Such tragedies can be easily prevented. Never leave your child in an unattended car, even with the windows down (many states have laws making it illegal to leave children alone in cars). If you're exhausted, stressed, or distracted, you can make mistakes you wouldn't otherwise make, especially if you're a new parent. To jog your memory, put your purse or cell phone in the backseat to remind you that your child is there. Or place a child's item, such as the diaper bag, in the front seat to remind you of the baby in the back.

Drowning: A Common Threat

With swimming pools and lakes so common in Florida, I see far too many kids who are the victims of accidental drownings. When children of any age are around water, they have to be watched and supervised by an adult every second. Infants and small children can drown in only a few inches of water.

One of the most dangerous scenarios I see occurs when a bunch of kids are playing in the water together and there is some roughhousing. I remember one situation in which a child was splashing around in the pool with other kids, and he got trapped underneath a raft. No one noticed, despite the pool being surrounded by adults; he ended up at the bottom of the pool, dead. To keep your own kids safe from drowning, never for a moment leave them unattended in a bath, swimming pool, wading pool, hot tub, or near any body of water, even a small bucket.

Keep Kids Safe from Guns

Accidental shootings take the lives of roughly two hundred children in the United States each year. I've handled a number of cases involving kids and guns. Once, in a heart-piercing case where child's play turned deadly, I had a nine-month-old baby who had been killed by his five-year-old brother. The five-year-old had climbed onto his parents' dresser where there was a loaded gun within easy reach. Not understanding what he was doing, the child grabbed the gun, pointed it at his little brother, and pulled the trigger.

The best way to prevent injury and death from firearms is to avoid keeping guns in your home and avoid exposing your children to households where guns are kept. If you do own a firearm, or the parents of your children's playmates do, protect your children by making sure guns are stored in a securely locked case, out of children's reach. All firearms should be stored unloaded and in the uncocked position. Be sure to emphasize to children that guns are not toys and should never be played with.

Accidents Don't Have to Happen

When I see bodies that emerge out of careless accidents—a lapse in judgment, a moment of forgetfulness, a tired decision—I can't help thinking that it could have happened to anybody, even me. Working in forensics has helped me become more aware of the consequences of everyday actions. Of all the killers that assault health, accidents are the most preventable. Here are some general guidelines to consider:

- Educate yourself on how to properly operate appliances, tools, and other equipment. Read operating manuals carefully. Know the possible dangers and how to avoid them.
- Wear protective gear if an activity calls for it: safety glasses, helmets, sports gear, and the like.
- Make sure you have experience before you do an activity. For example, do you know how to pilot a motorboat? Are you a good swimmer?
- Be aware of your state of mind before engaging in an activity. Are you bored? Tired? Distracted? Stressed out? A bad mood or fatigue can impair your judgment.
- Evaluate the riskiness of your behavior. Many accidents are the result of thoughtless or reckless behavior, such as riding motorcycles without helmets, diving headfirst into bodies of water without knowing their depth, and using drugs and alcohol unwisely. Think before you act.
- Take classes in first aid and CPR.

There may be no escaping the dangers of everyday life, but I believe that with enough forethought and attention, we can anticipate the risks involved in certain activities. And having anticipated them, we have the power to change our behavior or modify our environment to reduce risks and prevent tragic misfortunes. Carelessness can kill us, but it can be stopped.

LIFE LESSONS: Lightning Can Strike in Fair Skies

Lightning can zigzag across the sky, and it doesn't have to be raining. A bolt of lightning can come out of the blue, literally—so it's a good idea to keep your eyes on the skies. People often ask me what a body looks like after being struck by lightning. One telltale sign is "arborization"—marks in a fernlike, branching pattern on the body. Lightning can stop your heart, and that's how most people die. If lightning does strike, take cover right away in an enclosed building or a car with the windows rolled up, and not under a tree or any tall, isolated shelter like a picnic pavilion. Some other lifesaving tips:

- Get away from water.
- Never stand near a tall tree or telephone pole during a bad storm. Because humans are 70 percent water, and therefore conduct electricity more efficiently than wood, the lightning may jump from the tree or pole to you.
- Don't use electrical appliances or telephones with cords, since lightning can follow electrical wires and phone lines right into your home.
- Drop all lightning targets such as golf clubs, tennis rackets, and other metal items.
- If you take shelter in a car, don't touch any of its metal parts.
- If the storm strikes so suddenly that you don't have time to get inside, lie down on the ground and curl up into a ball.

THE ODDS OF DYING FROM ...

Accident	Lifetime Possibility
Car crash	1 in 84
Assault by firearm	1 in 324
Hit by a car	1 in 631
Choking	1 in 1,173
Fire in a building	1 in 1,431
Fall, involving bed or furniture	1 in 4,870
Airplane crash	1 in 5,552
Exposure to excessive natural cold	1 in 5,576
Drowning in a swimming pool	1 in 6,031
Slipping, tripping, or stumbling	1 in 6,455
Exposure to excessive natural heat	1 in 16,680
Hornet, wasp, or bee sting	1 in 72,494
Lightning strike	1 in 81,949
Overexertion	1 in 96,658
Contact with hot tap water	1 in 125,655
Dog bite	1 in 139,617
Venomous snake or lizard bite	1 in 628,277
Fireworks discharge	1 in 1,884,832

Source: National Safety Council

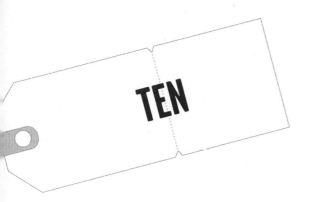

TEN

Man, Oh Man!

A Casualty of Impulse

While we do autopsies, music is playing in the morgue. One December morning, the music played "I'll Be Home for Christmas," a tune sadly unfitting for the four bodies lying in the autopsy suite. One of these was a twenty-nine-year-old decedent, now known as case number 88-1206. He was wheeled from the refrigerator into the autopsy suite, where my morgue assistant proceeded to undress the body. The dead man had long blond hair and was wearing a black T-shirt and a pair of jeans. Nothing but a cell phone and a wallet with thirty-three dollars in cash was found in his pockets. His driver's license identified him as Larry Andrews.

My technician began photographing the body. We rolled him over onto his stomach. I duly noted that there was a huge tattoo across the top of his buttocks. Tattoos often say something important about a person or tell me the identity of an unknown person. A military tattoo might give name, rank, and unit number. A Harley-Davidson tattoo is a sign the person was a biker. Some tattoos tell me the deceased had been in prison or in a gang. Tattoos might be anywhere on a body. I can't think of a place where I haven't seen a tattoo.

From the investigator's report and eyewitness accounts, I learned that this fellow had been at a card game the night before. At some point during the game, he stood up, uttered an expletive that in polite language means to have sexual intercourse, put a gun to his head, and pulled the trigger.

During the autopsy, I drew an enormous amount of clear liquid from his bladder into a syringe—a sign that he had been heavily intoxicated, which would later be confirmed by a toxicology report. His inebriation apparently set the stage for what looked like an impulsive act of suicide. I poked my gloved finger through his brain to determine the bullet's trajectory, from the point of entry behind his temple to the exit wound on the other side of his head.

More than thirty-two thousand suicides occur annually in the United States, according to the Centers for Disease Control—the equivalent of roughly eighty-eight suicides a day. Of those suicides, most are men. Men take their own lives at nearly four times the rate of women and thus represent nearly 79 percent of all suicides in the country. In fact, suicide is the eighth leading cause of death for men and the sixteenth leading cause of death for women.

But it's not only suicides that are taking the lives of so many men. They're dying from accidents at high rates, too. In the United States, accidents kill more than thirty-five thousand men every year—more than twice the rate of women. Astoundingly, for men between the ages of one and forty-four, accidents are the number one cause of death.

It isn't just the numbers that I find troubling, either. It's the kind of accidents men tend to fall victim to. Car crashes are the leading cause of accidental male death, and many are the result of driving aggressively and driving drunk. Men are more than three times as likely as women to drown, often as a result of stunts with speedboats and personal watercrafts. Some eight times as many men as women die mishandling firearms. Nine out of ten murderers—and eight in ten murder victims—are men.

Don't get me wrong; I'm not picking on men. But after working in the morgue for more than twenty years, I've observed a pattern that I think even my male colleagues would agree with: Men do stupid things. They drive aggressively or while under the influence, and they take risks involving boneheaded stunts and other behavior. And they pay with their lives, again and again.

Some choices men make are so dumb that I just have to believe they didn't take even a moment to think them through. For example, in one case of mine, a gentleman was helping a friend move a mattress. They didn't bring any rope to secure the mattress to the top of the car, so one of the guys decided to lie on top of it while they drove home. A mattress on top of a moving car is like a sail in the wind. Sure enough, less than a half mile into the transport, the mattress and the man were blown onto the road, and the man died. It was just plain goofy—and a senseless tragedy to boot.

Another time, I investigated the accidental death of a man who was attempting to fix something under his truck without using a jack. Instead, he drove his car up on a spare tire. The car rolled off the tire onto him, and he was killed instantly.

And if that isn't enough, men of all ages are experimenting with "car surfing." This involves standing on a car's hood, being towed on a skateboard, or hanging on a car's bumper while the car is cruising along at speeds up to fifty miles per hour or more. For anyone who chooses to car surf, just about every part of the body is at risk, especially the central nervous system. Serious injuries, such as head trauma, skull fractures, spinal cord injuries, and broken bones, or death, are distinct possibilities anytime someone goes car surfing. A lot of guys call it a sport; I call it another dumb stunt.

I've also handled cases like you'd see in a cartoon: A guy dies after sitting on a tree branch that he was sawing off. You hear a story like that and laugh at its stupidity, but the sad part is, someone died. I've thought about this for a long time and, frankly, I just don't see women doing these kinds of acts.

Men can be impressive in their tendency to self-destruct, explosively or gradually. What's the deal? Are men inherently more susceptible to accidents, suicides, and risk taking than women? If so, why? And what can be done about it?

The Alcohol Factor

Watery Grave

Several days dead and floating in a pond were enough to render this mystery man nearly unrecognizable. His flesh had turned mossy green and his body was unnaturally bloated. Dark purple veins marbled his chest. His skin had begun to separate from his hands, giving the illusion that he was wearing gloves complete with fingers—a process we medical examiners call "degloving." He still had dermal ridges on his fingertips, though, and fortunately could be fingerprinted for identification purposes.

Although he was definitely not easy on the eyes, the sight of this man did not compare to his overpowering stench. It was the smell of bodily gas, dead fish, rotten eggs, dirty underwear—well, you get the picture—and for many people, it's enough to make you surrender the contents of your stomach. The smell doesn't bother me, though—I guess I'm just used to it—but I wear hairspray, and since the smell tends to cling to hairspray, I cover my hair when examining a decomposing body.

After an autopsy like this, I change clothes so that I won't smell of corpse reek. Believe it or not, though, the odor of bodily decay may have value. Scientists have studied its composition so they can develop better synthetic sprays for possible use in riot control. I guess nothing breaks up a crowd like the smell of ripe decomp. And in our morgue, we save the rags used to clean up liquids from decomposed bodies to help train cadaver-hunting dogs.

Autopsying a decomposing body is a race against nature's grim clock. Once life has left it, the body begins a metamorphosis that involves two well-understood processes: autolysis and putrefaction. Autolysis is the breakdown of cells and organs by enzymes within a few hours of death. Putrefaction occurs as the result of bacterial action sweeping through the body. Bacteria convert soft tissue to liquids and gases, and the body begins to swell as a result of the trapped gases. The rate of decomposition depends on a number of factors, including the size of the body, ground conditions, and the temperature of the environment. Bacteria need warmth to grow—which is why you decompose faster in Florida than you do in Minnesota.

But back to the mystery man. On a March afternoon, a passerby saw a body floating facedown in a retention pond near an Orlando highway and immediately called police and EMS, who rushed to the scene. The retention pond itself was a three-foot-deep pool designed to collect rainwater. A paramedic waded out to his waist to recover the body and pulled it ashore. A call went out to my morgue, and we dispatched an investigator to the scene.

Near the edge of the retention pond, amid a dense forest of low-lying palms, was a makeshift shelter. Inside was a mattress and shelving filled with neatly stacked clothes and personal effects, including several bottles of mouthwash and a wallet with an ID belonging to a man named Robert Fowler. But whether the man in the pond was Robert Fowler was unclear.

Was this a death by drowning? Drowning deaths can be difficult to determine. I have to ask lots of questions. For instance, did the victim drown, or did perpetrators kill the individual and dump the corpse in the water? Was the victim conscious upon submersion? Could the person swim well? Did the victim consume any alcohol or drugs? What was the individual doing at the time? Did anyone witness the incident? If any injuries exist on the body, were they caused before death, at the same time, or afterward? Any evidence that can help answer such questions has to be gathered.

Initially, the body of a drowning victim sinks to the bottom of a lake, river, or pool. At some point later, the corpse eventually surfaces because of the gas formed in its tissues. In warm and shallow water like this retention pond, a corpse will rise to the surface in a day or two. In deep and cold water, bacterial action takes place more slowly, and the corpse may not surface for several weeks, and in very cold water, not at all. As for this body, I estimated that it had been in the water under the hot Florida sun for over a day and had definitely begun to decompose.

In an autopsy of a possible drowning victim, I look to see if the lungs are large and bulky, or if there's white foam in the trachea and bronchi. The stomach may contain water, too. Even so, no known and proven pathological test currently exists to determine drowning as the cause of death, so, by itself, an autopsy usually proves insufficient. I have to consider all the evidence collected at the scene and eliminate all other potential causes of death to make my diagnosis.

My first step was thus to make sense of what police officers and my investigator found at the scene. As I made annotations and measurements on diagrams attached to my clipboard, I noticed that despite the fact he was living in a tent, this man didn't look like a typical transient. His head was shaved, and his beard was well kempt. Then there was the mouthwash that was discovered in the tent. I don't know too many transients who use mouthwash. I didn't see any signs of trauma on him, but the internal examination might tell a different story.

Once I was inside the chest cavity, my challenges mounted. Because of the decomposition, his body fat had begun to liquefy like melting butter, and I had to be careful. I could easily cut myself, because the fat made my tools so slippery. One of the biggest problems, however, was that the major arteries were filled with air instead of blood. That's because blood decays faster than skin, muscles, or internal organs, so I couldn't draw any blood for toxicology. Partially decomposed organs could still show the presence of alcohol or drugs, although the results might be inconclusive.

It was only when I cut open his stomach to examine the contents that I got a tantalizing and unusual clue: His stomach contents smelled like mouthwash! I wondered if he had swilled mouthwash to get drunk. Several mouthwash products are fairly high in alcohol. It's not uncommon for alcoholics to drink alcohol-based products such as mouthwash and aftershave to reach high levels of intoxication. The bottles of mouthwash found in his tent contained 27 percent alcohol; they may not have been for personal hygiene after all.

As I continued the internal exam, I could find no evidence of natural disease or trauma. There was a lot I ruled out, but not a lot that I ruled in. My next clues would have to come from toxicology tests.

Two days after I performed the autopsy, our fingerprint experts confirmed his identity. The man in the retention pond was Robert Fowler, as the ID in the wallet suggested. He was a fairly young man—only thirty-five years old—and according to a college friend who came forward, Robert was not a typical transient. He was a bright, trained musician from a middle-class family in Oregon but unable to hold a job because of a drinking problem. Robert had confided in his friend that he also had bipolar disorder and that he was unable to overcome the obstacles of his illness. It was like a battle he fought and eventually lost. Robert took refuge in his homemade tent at the retention pond and settled into a way of life that seemed to satisfy him, away from mainstream society. Very little of this, however, explained how he wound up facedown in the water.

Toxicology tests on Robert's liver revealed a high level of alcohol in his system, but that finding wasn't reliable because of the advanced state of decay. When bacteria in the body run loose during decomposition, one of the materials they produce is alcohol. This meant that the test results didn't necessarily prove anything about his blood alcohol level. In the end I had to fall back on the one solid clue I discovered during the autopsy: the mouthwash in Robert's stomach.

With that in mind, this is what I believed happened: On the day of his death, Robert consumed a large amount of mouthwash. Either restless or possibly because his bladder was full, he stumbled from his tent toward the retention pond. He was intoxicated and fell into the water. I ruled his death an accidental drowning, since there was no evidence of trauma, natural disease, or other cause of death.

Guzzling mouthwash, though crazy, or throwing back a few drinks with the guys may seem harmless enough. But the statistics on men and alcohol reveal a disturbing relationship. Although exact figures may vary, studies indicate that men are at least twice as likely as women to be alcoholics and three times more likely to be drug addicts. Many male settings, from military units to college fraternities, encourage men to abuse alcohol as a rite of passage. Cirrhosis of the liver, a medical condition highly associated with chronic alcohol abuse, is twice as likely to take the lives of men than women.

Alcoholic abuse and masculinity seem to go hand in hand. Alcohol impairs judgment, and it slows the processing of information. Alcohol makes men feel invincible and is a big factor in accidental deaths.

Drinking was also the central issue in a case I worked on several years ago, involving two men, a cliff, and a case of beer. Two guys went on a camping trip. Even though there was a clearly visible sign that said "Do not camp within fifty feet of the cliff," that's exactly where they pitched their tent. Then they decided to have a few beers. After drinking, one guy had to relieve himself, so he got out of the tent, took a few steps in the dark, and plunged over the edge of the cliff to his death. That's probably why the park didn't want people putting their tents up near the cliff. Obviously, these guys didn't think about that.

But alcohol isn't the sole culprit in the high death rate for males. There's something else: their hormones.

The Testosterone Factor

Men are more likely to engage in risk-taking behaviors of all sorts, and a big part of the reason is the male hormone testosterone. Young men are the greatest risk takers. The peak of their risky behavior correlates closely with the peak of their testosterone production. By age fifty, men take fewer risks than they did at age nineteen. Not coincidentally, their testosterone levels are much lower at fifty, too.

Originally designed to equip men with an instantaneous burst of power—indispensable for staring down a wooly mammoth or swimming across a raging river for food in Stone Age times—testosterone profoundly affects physique, behavior, competitiveness, aggression, mood, and sexual drive. Fundamentally, testosterone is what makes a man a man. It deepens his voice, grows hair on his face, and strengthens his muscles.

Testosterone is also correlated with psychological dominance. Put two men in a room together, and the one with more testosterone will tend to dominate the interaction. Over millennia, men with higher levels of testosterone were the ones most favored by women and therefore most likely to produce offspring and perpetuate society. Men have ten to twenty times more testosterone than women. This is why it makes perfect sense not to have coed sports.

You might think your boyfriend, husband, or son is a careless, impulsive male—and you'd be right, sort of. But they probably can't help themselves. They're wired, partly by testosterone, to crave a certain amount of risk and be more attracted to thrill-seeking activities, such as hunting or drag racing. They're also more prone to self-destructive behavior—heavy drinking, risky sex, fighting, committing crimes, or driving dangerously—that might deliver them to my morgue.

But for me, testosterone, like alcohol, tells only part of the story. Why more men die in accidents or from suicides than women also has a lot to do with how men are raised.

The Social Factor

Society is also to blame—with "macho" conditioning that rewards men for taking risks and tackling danger head-on. Males may engage in risky behavior because of widely accepted and continually reinforced social norms.

The phenomenon of men behaving badly starts very early. Young boys are encouraged to play rough, take risks, and do more exciting things, whereas girls, at least in our culture, are brought up to be more cautious and more fearful. We protect little girls much more than we protect little boys. Parents are forever telling their daughters, "Don't do that; you're going to get hurt." Perhaps as a result, I don't see a lot of women in the morgue who have died from stupid accidents.

Men are also encouraged to hide their feelings and be less emotional. This may explain higher suicide rates for men than for women. Women tend to discuss their feelings, seek feedback, and take advice—and are more likely to tell their doctors how they feel. As a result, women get better treatment for depression and anxiety than men.

I have two boys, and I'm very cognizant of the fact that our society encourages showy displays of bravado, aggression, and daring. But I try to teach my sons to think about the consequences of their actions. Many accidents can be avoided if you just think a situation through.

LIFE LESSONS: Leading Causes of Death in Men

All Males, All Ages	Percent
1. Heart disease	27.2
2. Cancer	24.3
3. Unintentional injuries (accidents)	6.1
4. Stroke	5.0
5. Chronic lower respiratory diseases	5.0
6. Diabetes	3.0
7. Influenza and pneumonia	2.3
8. Suicide	2.2
9. Kidney disease	1.7
10. Alzheimer's disease	1.6

Source: Centers for Disease Control and Prevention

Risky Bedroom Behavior

As if accidents weren't enough, men's risk-taking behavior seems to extend to their sex lives. I suppose one of the most surprising and horrifying cases I ever autopsied was a man named Alex Chin. He lived his life as if nothing were wrong. But what I found at his autopsy unveiled his secret, a deadly disease that no amount of denial would ever change.

Sex, Lies, and Death

The story of how this thirty-six-year-old realtor came to my morgue began on March 17, 2004, when he fell ill after having dinner at home with two friends. Alex had recently separated from his wife, Reena.

Alex and Reena met eleven years ago and fell in love. Seven years of dating and four years of marriage, however, were marred by periodic breakups and fights. Finally, Reena filed for divorce.

On the night of the 17th, after his friends left, Alex spoke with Reena on the phone. He was feeling ill, and he didn't sound like himself. The call left her worried about his health.

The next morning, the Orlando police found Alex Chin dead in his apartment, cause of death unknown. Later that day, his body arrived at my morgue.

From what the police told me, emotional temperatures and suspicions had been running high among Alex's loved ones. They were fighting over who would get the body, even though the law is quite clear. Until the divorce was final, Reena had custody of Alex's remains. I told them to either get a lawyer or bury the hatchet with Reena. But it turned out that the family suspected that Reena had poisoned Alex.

He was pretty upset over the divorce, too. Could it have been suicide at the thought of losing Reena?

As I proceeded with the autopsy, I searched for external signs of suicide, such as scars from previous suicide attempts, but found none. Nor were there any signs of foul play, like a blow to the body or outward signs of strangulation.

Once I got to the internal examination, two things surprised me. The first surprise was his blood. Normally, after death, blood remains liquid. Alex's blood was heavily clotted, often a sign of a serious infection.

The second thing that surprised me was the condition of his lungs. They appeared to be infected, so I took a culture of the lung tissue for later analysis. I also selected small pieces of tissue to be processed onto slides.

Lungs are normally as light and airy as cotton candy, but Alex's were heavy and thick. Normal lungs weigh around 300 grams each; his weighed 1,050 grams. Alex Chin had been very sick. It looked like an extremely serious case of pneumonia, severe enough to have killed him.

Pneumonia is defined as any inflammation of the lungs that causes white blood cells and cellular debris to collect in the air sacs, a condition that interferes with breathing. Though usually treatable if caught in time, pneumonia is the leading cause of death from infection in the United States. There are more than fifty types of pneumonia, the most deadly of which are caused when the lungs are invaded by bacteria.

But why were Alex's lungs in such bad condition? Cultures of his lung tissue came back negative for bacterial pneumonia. Nothing yet explained what had happened to him. Nothing was making sense, until I studied the sections of his lung under the microscope.

What I saw was nothing short of shocking. Alex's pneumonia was a rare type, a type that only people who are immunosuppressed get. The kind of pneumonia that killed Alex Chin was caused not by an invading bacteria, but rather a common fungus that is usually harmless, easily kept in check by a healthy immune system. But if the immune system is weakened, the microbe can take hold in the lung's air sacs and reproduce in mass quantities. Millions of microbes and a fluid the body secretes in reaction to them fill the lungs. It turned out that Alex had Pneumocystis carinii pneumonia, the most common lung infection seen in AIDS patients.

Once I diagnosed this form of pneumonia, I ran other tests to see if he had AIDS, and those tests came back positive. After learning the painful truth about Alex and his disease, I immediately called his wife and told her that her husband's blood tested positive for HIV. The implications for his widow, who hadn't even realize he was sick, were staggering.

Finding that Alex had AIDS and had died of pneumonia came as a blow to Reena, who thought her husband was healthy—so healthy, in fact, that he rarely visited a doctor. To her knowledge, he had none of the most common risk factors for infection with HIV, the virus that causes AIDS. He wasn't gay, and he didn't use intravenous drugs. But after Reena's head cleared from the dreadful news, she recalled that during the last years of their marriage, he had frequently complained of minor respiratory symptoms and was treated for bronchitis.

To make matters worse, Reena received even more disturbing news later the same day: Alex knew he had AIDS. He had been diagnosed with HIV in 1994 through the health department. Alex apparently took none of the antiviral drugs that keep the disease at bay and prevent its development into full-blown AIDS. Nor did he take other drugs known to prevent major infections such as Pneumocystis carinii pneumonia. Instead, Alex pursued a series of less effective remedies. On the night of his death, Alex Chin, with his severely crippled immune system, lay down in his bed and passed away from AIDS-related complications.

Someone can be infected with HIV for years before developing symptoms. During this time a person may appear perfectly healthy. But any infected individual, whether or not he or she is feeling or looking well, is able to spread the virus to another person.

In thinking about this case, I'm sure many people have secrets they find difficult to confess even to themselves, let alone to others. The coping mechanisms that we use to deal with our problems are as complicated as the conditions they help us handle. Most patients with a fatal disease deny it at first, then gradually come to accept their conditions.

But rather than accept the unacceptable, Alex had chosen to deny the very existence of the disease and keep it a secret, perhaps because of the sheer psychological burden of living with the virus circulating within him. He had known about his condition for many years but had ignored the risks that unprotected sexual relations with his wife would bring. I know that denial can be a normal phase of coping with illness—and I sometimes wonder how I would handle living with the specter of a life-threatening illness—but Alex's risk-taking behavior seems almost homicidal. There's no excuse for his actions. He put his—and his wife's—life on the line.

For Reena, there was one last test to perform. She had to see if she had managed to have years of sexual relations with an HIV-infected man without becoming infected herself.

Reena immediately went to a clinic for an HIV test and returned after a long weekend of fear and prayer to hear the results. Luckily, the test results came back negative. Since her first negative result, Reena has been tested five times. Each time the result has been negative. While a long-term intimate partner has a moderate risk of contracting HIV, viruses can be unpredictable. Reena was lucky. It is as happy an ending as such a story might have.

How Not to Die If You're a Guy

If a man's proclivity for risky behavior—or perhaps "recklessness" is the better term—is wired into him, is trying to save him a lost cause? Not at all. I believe it's a matter of consciousness-raising: getting men to start thinking about risk and devising interventions to keep them from doing crazy stunts, driving drunk, having unsafe sex, or engaging in other Neanderthal-like behavior.

Here's my advice to men:

- Choose sports or physical exercises that channel your competitive drive.
- Learn responsible use of automobiles, motorcycles, and other vehicles, and good driving skills.
- Everybody has an internal gauge of danger, including guys. Listen to it, and don't put your—or others'—lives at risk. Just one millisecond of a screw-up on your part when driving, operating machinery, or working around the house, and you'll be one of the male statistics this year.
- Avoid the use and abuse of destructive substances. Tobacco, alcohol, and illicit drugs have a range of deleterious effects on the body. Alcohol is known to be associated with about one-third of suicides. It is a key factor in accidents of all types and plays a role in many homicides.
- Get an annual checkup and listen to your doctor. You understand your need for tuning your car's engine on a regular basis, and you're careful to buy new tires before the treads become paper-thin, but your attitude toward your body might be one of benign neglect. I've seen men live with medical problems until they escalate beyond easy management. An

illness that could have been treated without difficulty if caught early is allowed to become serious, even life-threatening.

- Be a responsible sexual partner. To avoid the risk of HIV infection, AIDS, and other sexually transmitted diseases, stick to one faithful partner, or at least use a condom to help protect yourself from potentially deadly infections.

- Take care of your emotional and mental health. It's important to have a social network of good friends who can sustain you in times of crisis, especially in times of loss and grief.

- Don't be shy about seeking professional help if you feel depressed, and that means feeling lousy, empty, unmotivated, or detached from the people around you. Men are reluctant to acknowledge these feelings, because there's a stricture that says depression is unmanly and a sign of weakness. Part of the reason for male resistance to seeking medical help may lie in our culture's expectations. Traditionally, boys are trained to keep their feelings under wraps. Self-reliance and toughness are valued. Real men don't get down and are expected to bear up under adversity. But trust me, real men do suffer from depression, and that's okay because there is help available, from friends, family, and from the medical community. There's nothing wrong with getting treatment, and the best is often a combination of psychotherapy (talk therapy) and antidepressant medication.

- Have a sense of purpose to your life beyond your occupation—a passion, something that guides you, be it love of a sport, a child or grandchild, books, or a social cause.

TURN THE TABLES: How to Live Past Ninety If You're a Man

A recent study published in the *Archives of Internal Medicine* looked at what characteristics define men who live longer than ninety years. Five behaviors jumped out at researchers: These men didn't smoke, exercised regularly, avoided diabetes, controlled their weight, and kept their blood pressure in check.

Men will be men, and much is beyond fixing. They're going to do reckless things, drive fast, and sometimes turn to aggression to cope with their anger and frustration. They just need to balance these traits with common sense. Let me add that other masculine traits, such as their take-charge attitude, leadership abilities, and protective nature, are admirable and why we love them so much.

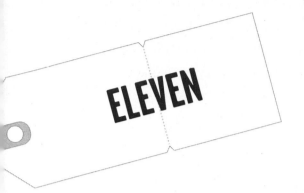

ELEVEN

Permanent Vacation

Economy Executioner

Every year, millions of tourists flock to the theme parks of Orlando, Florida, which happen to be near my morgue. Most people go on vacation—whether here or anywhere—to relax, unwind, and have fun with family and friends. But for a small, sad few, a vacation turns out to be their final act.

A few summers ago, a widowed seventy-three-year-old businessman from England, Julian Noble, flew four thousand miles to Orlando to visit his family, including his grandkids, who hadn't seen him in more than a year. From the moment his plane landed, he complained of abdominal pain that persisted through the next morning. At breakfast, Julian doubled over and collapsed. His son dialed 911. Within minutes, an ambulance crew arrived, and performed CPR on the way to the hospital, but they were not able to revive him. Julian died on the way.

Julian's son was desperate to know what had killed his father. It became my job to find out, and to piece together the story of this man's demise. Because Julian was from overseas, there was little background information available, making it difficult to narrow down the possible causes of death.

I began the autopsy by performing the external examination but found nothing of note after poring over every inch of his body. To begin the internal exam, I snapped a blade into a handle, and with strong strokes made a Y incision and cut through the skin to open up the whole torso. I focused first on the abdomen. Based on Julian's symptoms, I considered several conditions that might have killed him so quickly: an infarcted bowel, diverticulitis, or an abdominal aortic aneurysm.

First, I looked at his intestines for infarcted bowel, which is a belly with a dead bowel in it. When blood doesn't get to the bowel for some reason, parts of it die. I inspected Julian's bowel, looking for signs of dead tissue. But once again, I found nothing out of the ordinary.

Next, I examined Julian's colon to look for signs of diverticulitis, a potentially lethal condition of the colon often associated with a low-fiber diet and lack of exercise. This condition begins as diverticulosis, the presence of pockets or protrusions in the wall of the colon. When these sacs become inflamed and infected, the condition is termed diverticulitis. Then you can become quite ill—with fever, cramps, and on occasion, blood in the stools. Diverticulitis can sometimes lead to a perforation of the bowel. If Julian had diverticulitis, I would find the telltale signs of infection in his abdominal cavity—free fluid or pus. But after a thorough exam, I came up empty.

I searched Julian's abdominal cavity for signs of an aneurysm. An abdominal aneurysm develops when the aorta, which runs from the heart through the abdomen, becomes weakened and balloons out due to atherosclerosis, the buildup of cholesterol plaque in blood vessels. This weakened area can eventually leak or rupture—and that's a life-threatening emergency. When that happens, blood rushes into the abdominal cavity, and the victim swiftly dies from internal bleeding. But there was no free blood in the abdominal cavity. He hadn't died from an aortic aneurysm.

Pressing on for answers, I examined the rest of his abdominal cavity, inch by inch, eventually coming to the gallbladder. Roughly the size of an apricot, the gallbladder sits just beneath the liver. Its job is to store bile produced by the liver and secrete it whenever fat needs to be digested. Here, I got my first clue. Julian's gallbladder was inflamed and thickened. When the gallbladder is acutely inflamed, it's usually because stones—crystallized clumps of fatty material or bile pigment—have accumulated inside it. As I sliced through the gallbladder, I immediately found gallstones. These gallstones may have been the cause of Julian's abdominal pain, but the question was, did they kill him?

Gallstones are a common condition that affects one in ten adults in America and Europe. Most people who have gallstones don't feel any symptoms. However, your first awareness might come from mild pain in the pit, or upper right part of your belly. The pain may spread to the back near your right shoulder blade. Sometimes the pain is severe, or it may come and go or get worse when you eat. If the stones are small enough, you'll usually pass them. But if the stones become lodged in the ducts that carry bile to the intestines, you'll have to have them removed.

In my experience, gallstones are rarely fatal and, at first glance, it appeared that they did not cause Julian's death. However, gallstones can kill you by causing pancreatitis, an inflammation of the pancreas. If gallstones get stuck in the bile duct, they can block the flow of digestive juices through the tubes that lead from the pancreas. The pancreas will start digesting itself, and you can die.

I lifted up the stomach and liver to view the pancreas. It looked normal. I began to wonder whether Julian's abdominal pain was completely unrelated to his death. With this thought in mind, I next removed Julian's heart and examined it for coronary artery disease. Arteries clogged by cholesterol look yellow, sometimes in small areas of the vessel, other times throughout the vessel.

When I saw his heart up close, I was amazed by the healthy shape it was in. I will be so lucky if at seventy-three my coronaries look that clean. I could find no anatomic reason for that heart to have killed him. So far I had no clues as to why he died. I felt as though I were fishing, tossing a net out in the hopes that I'd somehow catch his killer.

I removed Julian Noble's lungs—one of my last hopes for finding a cause of death—and dissected them, looking for any anomaly. Surprise, surprise. Diagnostically, I went from crawling in the dark to sprinting in the sunlight. I found blood clots in both the right and left main pulmonary arteries. Those were his killers.

Since the vast majority of pulmonary blood clots form in the legs, I next dissected the backs of his legs. Sure enough, lurking in Julian's leg veins were clots, parts of which had broken away. When a piece of a clot breaks off and gets swept from the leg into the vena cava—the vein that carries deoxygenated blood into the heart's right chamber—and on into a lung, it can lodge in a lung vessel, blocking blood flow. Large pulmonary clots, as I found in Julian's case, can cause you to die suddenly and usually without warning. The blood is blocked from going into the lungs, and thus no blood can get to the heart to pump. A clot in the lung can be as lethal as it is elusive. Technically, Julian died as a result of an affliction known as deep vein thrombosis (DVT), often brought on by hours of immobility in an airplane.

The story of what happened to Julian Noble was now clear to me. While he was on the plane, a clot formed in his legs. The next morning, two large pieces of that clot traveled to his lungs and lodged in the pulmonary arteries, obstructing blood flow. Julian's heart, deprived of oxygen-rich blood, ceased to beat, and he died. Traveling can bring with it a host of occasional but catastrophic dangers, and Julian Noble had succumbed to one of them.

How Not to Die on Vacation

Bad things can happen to anyone on vacation. I'd be the last person, however, to advise you not to take a vacation. We all know about the negative impact of stress on the body; sometimes not taking some time away can be a dangerous proposition.

The word "vacation" means to empty yourself of work and pressures, replacing them with leisure and refreshment. Traveling is often a great break from the ordinary routine, and with the right planning, a vacation can be the relaxing escape it was meant to be. By packing some common sense, you can make sure that you're doing everything you can to stay safe and well on your next trip.

The Clot Thickens

With flight times now exceeding the gestation periods of some birds, there have been growing concerns about DVT, the cause of Julian Noble's death and a hidden danger I see several times a year in travelers.

DVT has been dubbed "economy class syndrome," reflecting the cramped legroom in economy class airline seating. But it can happen to passengers in any seating class of an aircraft. It can also happen on long rides in cars, trains, or buses, or even after you've sat at your desk all day.

Usually the body is able to naturally break up clots that form in the bloodstream, but with immobility, the blood becomes sluggish, and clots form that the body can't dismantle. Once the person gets up from his or her seat and is mobile again, a clot may break off and travel to the lungs.

I'm not one to splurge on luxury seats, so I fly economy class. After what I've seen, I always make sure I drink plenty of fluids to prevent dehydration. Dehydration causes blood to thicken, increasing the risk for DVT. I also get up every half hour or so to move and stretch my legs. I do exercises in my seat, like contracting and relaxing my legs. Many of the in-flight magazines contain instructions on how to perform exercises in your seat. A two-hour flight might not be a problem, but a twelve-hour flight could be if you're inactive the entire time. Children who travel aren't usually at risk for DVT, partly because they are generally more active in their seats than adults are.

There are other precautions that can minimize your risk of DVT. Even while waiting in the airport terminal, it's important to keep moving your legs to help blood flow. Get up and walk around when you can. When you walk, the muscles of the legs squeeze the veins and move blood to the heart. If you can't walk around in the plane or terminal, exercise your legs by curling or pressing your toes down. This causes the muscles to contract and squeeze on the leg veins, helping to pump the blood along.

When traveling by car, try to stop every couple of hours. Get out and walk a bit. Even if you're the driver, you still need to take walking breaks. Pushing on the gas pedal isn't enough activity even for the one leg.

Although DVT and the resulting blood clots don't usually broadcast their symptoms, warning signs may include chest pain, unexplained shortness of breath, ankle swelling, tenderness, or a warm feeling in the calf of one leg. These can appear during a very long trip or within a couple of days after flying. If you experience any of these symptoms, seek medical attention. There isn't much value in putting your feet up or drinking lots of water at this point. Getting medical help quickly is your best shot.

Protect Against the Number One Vacation Killer

Here's something that may surprise you: The most common cause of death while traveling is heart attack, and it usually strikes within the first couple of days of a vacation, mainly in people with heart trouble. I've autopsied many travelers with weak hearts who succumbed to sudden cardiac death, even though they were often walking, talking, and feeling fine when it struck.

A Heart-Stopping Trip

The last day of Martin Landers's life began with planning which tourist attractions in Orlando he and his wife would visit on their vacation. Their first—and final—stop would be at one of the city's many water parks. One of the fifty million visitors to Orlando annually, Martin, age fifty-five, was a stout 375 pounds. At the water park, Martin began climbing the stairs of a large waterslide, one advertised to blast riders down a tube at twenty-five miles per hour. He turned to his wife, who was just behind him, and told her, "I'm not feeling too well. My chest hurts." Yet he continued the ride anyway. At the bottom of the slide, he collapsed and went into cardiac arrest.

Lifeguards responded immediately, began CPR on Martin, and called an ambulance. Paramedics scrambled to hook him up to a portable cardiac unit. They grabbed two defibrillating paddles and pushed one against Martin's upper chest and the other against his left rib cage. If all went well, the electric current between the two paddles would flow through his heart and jump-start a normal electrical rhythm. The paramedics worked until there was nothing more to do. They could not bring back Martin's dying heart, and he wound up in my morgue.

When someone dies at an amusement park, stories in the media often give the impression that the ride or the park was at fault. This is rarely the case. The death investigation of Martin Landers, for example, revealed that he had a pre-existing heart condition. Overexerting himself brought on the heart attack. The waterslide had nothing to do with his death.

It seems a cruel twist of fate to go on vacation to relax and shut out the stresses of everyday life, only to be stricken by a heart attack. But often when people are on vacation, they tax their bodies by doing things they're not normally accustomed to doing. They may be overly active, or they may overreact to some of the normal stresses of traveling. Any abrupt, accelerated change in behavior can trigger a heart attack, particularly in someone with cardiac risk factors, such as high blood pressure, diabetes, smoking, high cholesterol, or a family history of early heart disease.

My advice boils down to basic common sense. Be careful what you do on vacation. If you try to cram in a lot of activities you're not used to doing, you can put yourself at a higher risk for heart attacks or other problems. Take it easy on your trip, and you'll have a better vacation.

People who feel sick on vacation often don't seek prompt medical attention. It's unfamiliar territory and they don't know where to go or who to call, so they think they'll ride it out. They don't want their vacation spoiled. If you're on vacation and start to feel ill, please don't ignore unusual symptoms. Get checked out as soon as possible. What's the worst thing that can happen if you're wrong about your symptoms? You'll find out you're fine and get to resume your vacation.

If you're going to be traveling to a foreign country, plan ahead. Get a free list of English-speaking doctors in many countries around the world from the International Association for Medical Assistance to Travelers at www.iamat.org; or (716) 754-4883. Otherwise, you can usually find English-speaking doctors by contacting the staff at a large hotel or the local U.S. consulate or embassy.

Thrills Without Spills

Part carnival, part thrill show, tantalizing with the aroma of popcorn and hot dogs and exhilarating with bright lights and squeals of delight, amusement and theme parks pulse with a sense of controlled terror. The sheer outrageousness of some of the rides—roller coasters that plunge at megaspeeds, whirligigs that make your stomach flutter, space-age capsules that flip their occupants upside down—adds to the excitement.

When you go to an amusement park, you're invited to check your worries at the ticket gate. And, statistically speaking, that invitation is an honest one. The chance of having an injury resulting in death at an amusement park is less than one in fifty million, making this industry one of the safest in the world.

Sadly, though, I do a few autopsies each year of people, young and old, who die at the area's theme parks. Like the case of Martin Landers, it's seldom the ride that kills them, but the state of their health, known or unknown. Another time, a forty-seven-year-old Austrian tourist, Greta Petersen, was hospitalized after going on an attraction that spins riders at three times the earth's gravity. After the ride ended, she complained of dizziness, one side of her face was drooping, and she was rushed to the hospital. A CAT scan of her brain prompted doctors at the hospital to conclude that Greta had suffered a "bleed within the brain," in other words, a stroke.

A stroke is the brain's version of a heart attack. There are two main kinds. One is caused by a clot in a blood vessel of the brain. The other is caused when a brain blood vessel ruptures and blood leaks into brain tissue, and this is the type Greta had. Both disrupt the oxygen flow in the brain, often causing permanent brain damage if you live. If the stroke is of great magnitude, you can't walk without assistance; you can't bathe; you can't dress. Greta Petersen died about twenty-four hours after being admitted to the hospital.

The autopsy is an important tool for determining the cause of death, but.it has to be taken in the context of other information supplied. Clues are found in the patient's history and information from the scene of a death. From reading her history and my investigator's report, I learned that Greta had decided not to take her blood pressure medication. She had passed out several days earlier but chose not to see a doctor. I related this information to my findings from the autopsy, which confirmed several things. First, she did have a hypertensive bleed in her brain. Second, she had severe, long-standing high blood pressure, which I could see evidence of in the blood vessels of her brain and in her heart. And third, she had suffered a smaller stroke several days earlier. Greta's days were numbered because her high blood pressure was not being aggressively treated.

Every time I have a death associated with one of the many amusement park rides here in Orlando, I get letters and e-mails letting me know how dangerous g-forces are, and that it is the dangerous g-forces that must have done the person in. A "g-force" is a measurement of the gravitational stress on the body undergoing rapid acceleration. One g, for example, is the acceleration of normal earth gravity. This acceleration can be in a vertical (up and down), horizontal (forward or backward), or lateral (side to side) direction. That's what makes a roller coaster fun. Human tolerance to acceleration depends on the magnitude of the acceleration, the direction, the rate of onset, and the duration of acceleration. Sustained accelerations (those lasting longer than .2 seconds) will shift body fluids and cause physiologic effects, thus making your heart work harder. High enough g-forces will cause blackouts; higher still, even for a moment, will cause death.

Even the most exhilarating amusement park rides tend to create g-forces of 3 or less and only for short periods of time. A few roller coasters have been stated to feature 4 g's and, possibly a few in the world measured at 5 g's but, again, only briefly. Keep in mind that during everyday events we experience g-forces for short periods of time. A cough is estimated to be 3.5 g's and hopping off a step as high as 8 g's. Pilots routinely endure 8 or 9 g's.

Greta rode on an attraction that subjects riders to three times the normal force of gravity. Most people can withstand these forces. However, if you have hypertension, low blood sugar, heat stress, infections, or are dehydrated or under the influence of alcohol, your body's tolerance of g-forces will be much lower, and you can become ill. If you've got a physical condition, such as a bad back or a weak heart, that might be exacerbated by a ride, stay off.

The culture of amusement parks seems to foster bad choices and behavior—and accidents. The lights, the noise, and the feeling of recklessness all raise the stakes. People, especially kids, do crazy things. Horseplay, not paying attention to the warnings, disrupting a ride—these are what cause most accidents that I see in the morgue. Yet they are avoidable.

I rode a roller coaster recently with my son at a local amusement park. As soon as we were seated, the announcer cautioned us to brace our heads against the headrest while the ride was moving. You can bet that mine was pressed very tightly against that headrest, and well secured. Always pay attention to such announcements, as well as to posted warnings such as: "For safety you should be in good health and free from high blood pressure; heart, back, or neck problems; motion sickness; or other conditions that can be aggravated by this adventure."

Adhere to all the rules. Follow all weight, height, and age restrictions to the letter. Once on board, keep your hands and arms in the car and hold on to the safety bar. Then relax and have fun. Amusement parks are safe, especially when you're safety minded.

Don't Go Near Dangerous Waters

During warm weather, police radios in Orlando crackle with reports of people who have just drowned. Accidental drownings seem to peak during the spring and summer in my jurisdiction. This is the time when tourists come to Orlando with their kids, and they are not used to the extreme attention needed to watch children around pools. Often, families rent vacation homes and condos with pools, and people aren't used to having a pool around and don't know its risks. You and your family can have fun and still be safe around water by following the guidelines I've listed on page 226. In addition, when planning outdoor water activities, select areas that have good water quality and safe natural conditions. Murky water and aquatic plant life can be hazardous, as I learned in the strange case of fifteen-year-old Adam Camp in the summer of 2007.

Microbe Murderer

At first, it seemed like nothing more than a headache. But Adam continued to get sicker. He lapsed into a coma and was taken to an Orlando emergency room, where he died. Initially, the ER staff thought he had meningococcal meningitis, a contagious and often fatal infection.

As I examined Adam's brain during the autopsy, I was able to easily determine that the boy had indeed died from some sort of brain infection. But when I went looking for the underlying cause, I was surprised that none of the usual suspects—such as bacteria—were present.

Weeks later, I got my first look at the brain tissue under the microscope. I immediately saw an amoeba. I took samples to two other local pathologists to verify my suspicion. When they agreed with me, I alerted the Orange County Health Department. Initially, they were skeptical that I had tied Adam's death to an amoeba infection, and we sent samples to the CDC for further analysis. Scientists there confirmed that the teen had died from a brain infection caused by freshwater amoebas.

Later that summer, two other boys were killed by the same unusual infection, which they contracted after swimming in lakes in Orange County, Florida: primary amoebic meningoencephalitis, a brain infection caused by an amoeba known as *Naegleria fowleri.* This amoeba is common in Florida and many parts of the world. It lives in the soil on the bottom of warm freshwater lakes, rivers, ponds, and hot springs, but it can also be found in unchlorinated swimming pools.

It sounds like science fiction, but it's true: A killer amoeba living in lakes enters the body through the nose when swimmers dive or jump into the water. It works its way into the brain. Early symptoms of an infection include headache, fever, vomiting, and a stiff neck. As the illness progresses, people become lethargic and confused. They might suffer seizures or become unconscious. Antibiotics can be used to fight the infection, but survival is rare. Once inside the body, the amoeba just divides and divides, attacking and feeding on the brain, until you die.

How had Adam Camp contracted this infection? His family said he had not been in any lakes or ponds in the days before he got sick. He had gone swimming in a pool at an apartment complex, but amoebas cannot survive in properly chlorinated water. Health inspectors went to the apartment complex and tested the water in all five of its swimming pools. The tests showed that the chlorine levels were fine and that the water was not infested with amoebas.

This illness is extremely rare. There have been few documented cases in the United States. The Florida Department of Health counts only fourteen cases—including the three in 2007—during the past three decades.

Water Safety Tips

- Avoid alcohol and drug use before and during activities in or around water or while supervising children.
- Choose swimming areas that are supervised by trained and certified lifeguards and obey all rules, posted signs, and warning flags.
- Rip currents are a deadly ocean occurrence. The best way to get out of a rip current is to float on your back until the current stops pulling you, then swim parallel to the shore until you are past the current, then return to shore. Never swim directly into the current.
- If you don't know the water depth, avoid diving; a feetfirst entry is safer than headfirst.
- Wear a properly fitted personal flotation device (life jacket or vest) when boating, water skiing, or using a personal watercraft, regardless of the distance to be traveled, the size of the craft, or your swimming ability.
- If planning to scuba dive, obtain appropriate training and certifications, heed safety recommendations, and learn the signs and symptoms of decompression illness (joint pain, rash, numbness or tingling, weakness, paralysis, impaired thinking, shortness of breath or coughing, and dizziness or loss of balance).

In the end, the case of Adam Camp leaves us with a puzzle and a warning. The puzzle is how he had come into contact with the amoeba. Forensic investigations often fail to find an actual smoking gun, but we can still reach valid conclusions. The warning is to be especially cautious in all freshwater bodies, which pose a risk when water temperatures reach eighty degrees and above. The best way to prevent infection is to hold your nose or use nose plugs when jumping or diving into water. Stepping or walking into the water, rather than jumping or diving, may also help prevent the disease as well as other types of injuries.

A Shot at Health

Sixty-three million Americans travel overseas each year. If you're one of them and planning a trip to a foreign country, schedule a pre-trip checkup with a travel clinic at least four to six weeks before your departure. This is a must if you're traveling to the less-developed areas of the world, since most primary care physicians may not be familiar with the intricacies of travel medicine. Nonetheless, it's also important to check with your doctor to see whether any preexisting illness you have might be adversely affected by travel. Be sure to go over your immunization status, as well as any vaccines required for your destination country. Certain vaccines are recommended to protect travelers from illnesses present in other parts of the world and to prevent the importation of infectious diseases across international borders.

Which vaccinations you need depends on a number of factors, including your destination, whether you'll be spending time in rural areas, the season of the year you're traveling, your age and health status, and previous immunizations. My husband and I are planning a trip to Italy this year, for example, and the recommended vaccines for that country are routine shots such as the measles/mumps/rubella (MMR) vaccine and the diphtheria/pertussis/tetanus (DPT) vaccine. Anyone who is already up-to-date with their vaccinations wouldn't need them.

It's sometimes necessary to be vaccinated against specific illnesses: yellow fever, for example, for travel to certain countries in sub–Saharan Africa and tropical

South America; and meningococcal meningitis, which is required by the government of Saudi Arabia for annual travel during the hajj, a pilgrimage to the holy places of Islam, and recommended for several countries in central Africa. Depending on your itinerary, you may need vaccines for typhoid, hepatitis A, hepatitis B, Japanese encephalitis, or rabies.

If you're traveling to Africa, Central or South America, or Southeast Asia, take precautions to prevent malaria, a tropical disease that kills more than one million people a year, mostly infants, young children, and pregnant women. Every year, nearly 1,200 American travelers become severely ill with malaria.

Malaria is caused by a parasite called plasmodium, which is transmitted via the bites of infected mosquitoes. In the human body, the parasites multiply in the liver, and then infect red blood cells. Symptoms of malaria include fever, headache, chills, and sweats, and usually appear between ten days and six months after the mosquito bite. If not treated, malaria can quickly become life-threatening by disrupting the blood supply to your vital organs.

Malaria is both preventable and curable. Prevention involves avoiding mosquito bites and taking a preventive antimalarial drug when traveling to risky areas. Even the best malaria prevention is only about 95 percent effective, however, which is why you must be alert and seek medical help if you suffer from unexplained fever or unusual symptoms for up to a year after returning home.

A good source of information for required vaccinations and travel precautions outside the United States is the CDC at www.cdc.gov. This website also gives a list of locations for travel clinics in the United States.

Traveler's Curse

There's a saying that travel broadens the mind and loosens the bowels. The latter refers to traveler's diarrhea. Although it won't kill you, traveler's diarrhea can kill the fun of your vacation. Known as food poisoning, turista, or Montezuma's revenge, it's the number one illness afflicting vacationers, causing diarrhea, nausea, vomiting, stomach cramps, achiness, and fever. Areas with the highest risk include Mexico, South America, Africa, and parts of Asia.

Traveler's diarrhea is usually caused by bacteria (such as E. coli) and parasites found in food and water. Highly contagious viruses, such as noroviruses, are also potential culprits, especially on cruise ships, where they can spread rapidly via contact with infected travelers or contaminated food or water. Milder cases of turista can be chalked up to indigestion—from overindulgence or because you're not used to the food.

You can cut your risk by drinking only bottled water (even using it to brush your teeth), steering clear of ice cubes, and avoiding street-vendor foods. A rule of thumb when eating in exotic locales: If you can't peel it, boil it, or cook it, then forget it. And no matter where you go, eat and drink in moderation and wash your hands frequently.

If traveler's diarrhea strikes, be sure to consume plenty of salty fluids like chicken soup, or beverages with electrolytes such as Gatorade or Pedialyte, to replenish lost liquids and nutrients. If your symptoms are severe (accompanied by fever or bloody stools) or persist beyond a couple of days, you may need antibiotics, which are routinely provided as part of your travel clinic visit.

I can't overstate the importance of travel evaluation and counseling. The few hundred dollars it costs for counseling, vaccines, and preventive medications may save the trip of a lifetime or maybe even your life.

Passport to Health

When all is said and done, a vacation may actually save your life. Some research suggests that taking at least one vacation per year increases longevity by reducing the kind of stress that has been linked to heart attack, hypertension, depression, and other illnesses. And here is a whopper of an effect: A study done by psychologists and published in *Psychosomatic Medicine* showed that men who take more frequent vacations have a 30 percent lower risk of dying of heart disease, and women have a 50 percent less chance of dying of heart disease, compared to those who don't vacation.

There are a number of reasons why vacations can be good for your health. You're away from the stress and pressure of work. You get to relax. You have an opportunity to spend time with family and friends, hopefully in a positive environment.

Although I have to force myself to take vacations, I always enjoy them. It's fun to get a different perspective of the world and how people live. My family likes to unwind by enjoying a cruise, beachcombing, watching beautiful sunsets, experiencing new cuisines, and seeing different types of architecture. We enjoy spending this time together as a family. I purposely take off my watch during the week and try to plan as little as possible.

The only stress is when I come back. The case files, crime-scene reports, and toxicology results are stacked higher than when I left. Who sent all of these faxes, and why does the pile of phone messages look like the latest edition of the Orlando phone book? Oh well, only fifty-one weeks until my next vacation.

TURN THE TABLES: The Price of Passion

Yes, it's your vacation, and you're entitled to have a great time. But did you know that most sexually transmitted diseases (STDs) are diagnosed in late summer and autumn, as well as after Christmas? Medical experts blame vacation flings and risky sexual behavior on lowered inhibitions. Be smart. Before vacation, set your bedroom boundaries, and then stick to them.

Pack a Traveler's First-Aid Kit

For added safety, consider taking a first-aid kit with you on your next trip. What you pack depends on your destination, how long you'll be away, the type of travel, and any preexisting medical conditions you have. Here are some suggestions from the CDC:

Medications*:

- Personal prescription medications in their original containers (with copies of all prescriptions)

- Antimalarial medications, if applicable

- Over-the-counter antidiarrheal medication such as Pepto-Bismol

- Antihistamine

- Decongestant, alone or in combination with antihistamine

- Anti–motion sickness medication

- Acetaminophen, aspirin, ibuprofen, or other medication for pain or fever

- Mild laxative

- Cough suppressant/expectorant

- Throat lozenges

- Antacids

- Antifungal and antibacterial ointments or creams

- 1 percent hydrocortisone cream

- Epinephrine autoinjector (such as EpiPen) if you have history of severe allergic reaction

*Certain larger liquids such as medications, baby formula and food, breast milk, and juice can be placed in your carry-on luggage. These are allowed in reasonable quantities exceeding three ounces and are not required to be in a zip-top bag. Declare these items for inspection at the checkpoint.

Other important items:

- Insect repellent containing DEET* (up to 30 percent)

- Bed net if you're traveling to malaria-prone areas and not sleeping in a screened or air-conditioned room

- Sunscreen* (preferably SPF 15 or greater)

- Aloe gel* for sunburns

- Digital thermometer

- Basic first-aid items (adhesive bandages, gauze, ACE wrap, antiseptic, cotton-tipped applicators)

- Antibacterial hand wipes or alcohol-based hand sanitizer* containing at least 60 percent alcohol

- Moleskin for blisters

- Lubricating eye drops*

*If you place these items in your carry-on luggage, they'll need to be in three-ounce bottles or less (by volume) and put in one quart-sized, clear, plastic, zip-top bag.

Other items that may be useful in certain circumstances:

- Mild sedative or other sleep aid

- Antianxiety medication

- High-altitude-sickness preventive medication

- Water purification tablets

- Latex condoms

- Address and phone numbers of area hospitals or clinics

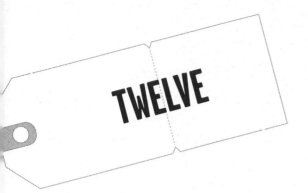
TWELVE

Longevity Rx

Since the advent of digital photography, I rarely visit the scene of a death, but during my early days as a medical examiner, I did. On a chilly March day in 1993, I entered the home of Mary Nance, a woman in her late fifties who had been found dead in her living room. What I saw stuck to my brain like superglue. Propped up in an armchair like an old doll with matted, messed-up hair was Mary Nance, staring but facing nothing, not even the television set in the room. Everywhere I looked, I saw clutter, feces, and cigarette ashes. The scent coming from the scene made me hold my breath. Death is sometimes ugly, and it can smell horrible.

I'll never know the whole story, but her estranged family told me that she didn't want to eat or leave her chair, even though she was quite capable of both. She had given up on life and was chronically depressed. She had nothing positive to focus on and no reason to get out of that chair. In some ways, she died long before she ever got to the morgue. Was hers a natural death? A suicide? You could call it either.

This gruesome image framed for me a picture of what happens when someone decides to sit out life, literally, and I'll never forget it.

I'm not afraid to admit that I have bad days—plenty of them. There's lots of busywork that consumes a big part of my week: lawyers to answer to, testimony to prepare, autopsy reports to write, and more. Sometimes I don't feel like doing anything except sitting around. Life can be a struggle, and there are daily challenges, both great and small, to overcome. For me, it's important to find purpose and order in life. I'm not about to become what I call "the woman in the chair."

I'm a strong believer that the mind and body are snugly interwoven, and this connection affects you in more ways than you might be aware. The mind and immune system, for example, don't exist independently of each other. Research shows that they act as a single unit. Feeling stressed can make you more susceptible to whatever bug is going around, and this is something I always keep in mind. If I get sick, I'm no good to anyone, so I do what I can to keep my stress to a minimum. When I worked in San Antonio, my kids were both young, and my then-husband and I had full-time medical careers. We were both going full steam, and I felt like something was going to fall apart. I worried it was going to be our marriage or family life. I decided to pull back from my morgue work and simplify my life. So I shared my job with another forensic pathologist, who also wanted to spend more time with her family. This arrangement calmed me down considerably.

Then there's depression, which increases your odds of dying from many medical causes. Depressed or angry people are less likely to stick with diet and exercise programs and are more likely to smoke or abuse alcohol and drugs. Sadly, I see what happens when depression either goes untreated or goes poorly treated for months or years. People sink into an emotional abyss so deep that they can't climb out and decide to kill themselves instead. Suicides are always the saddest cases, because you know the victims must have felt incredible anguish before they did it. I'll be the first to admit that life can get tough, but part of life is that you have to get up every day with something to live for and keep going.

People with depression are also more prone to heart disease, and people with heart disease are more likely to suffer depression. Consider these statistics from recent studies: Depressed patients with heart attacks are four times more likely to die within six months than are their nondepressed counterparts. Depressed people with newly diagnosed heart disease are twice as likely to have a heart attack or require bypass surgery. It's only natural to be down in the dumps about such a clear reminder of our mortality as heart disease, but treating the depression, as well as the disease itself, can help you get better. Why is there such a strong link between depression and heart disease? No one knows for sure, but when the nervous system (of which the brain is a part) has problems, the whole body has problems, including the heart.

Now for the flip side: Positive emotions are good for your health! When you feel joyous and lighthearted, your immune system has a better chance of protecting you from disease. Positive thinkers tend to take good care of themselves and have normal blood pressure. They tend to live longer, too. In a long-running study, Duke University researchers gave a personality test to more than seven thousand students. Each person was typed as either an optimist or a pessimist. During a forty-year follow-up period, optimists had increased longevity. The researchers explained their findings by saying that optimists don't usually suffer from depression, are more likely to use the health-care system to their benefit, follow healthy diets, and get regular exercise. I like to think that I'm a positive person most of the time, so I was glad to learn that my attitude may affect my longevity.

Happiness can help you live a longer, healthier life. A study from University College London showed that people who are happy and unstressed have lower levels of stress-associated chemicals in their bodies. One of these chemicals is cortisol, an essential hormone, which in excess is associated with abdominal obesity, type 2 diabetes, high blood pressure, and slow wound healing. The researchers also discovered that happy people have lower levels of the stress-induced substance plasma fibrinogen, which correlates with inflammation in the body and increased risk of heart disease and stroke. Happiness is good for the heart.

It bears mentioning that having more "things" does not bring happiness. I had somebody say to me just the other day, "Oh, I'm so jealous of your career and the amount of money you must make being a doctor." I was floored because the person in question is talented, healthy, the parent of two beautiful children, and has a lot going for her. Happiness is not about how much money you make.

Most psychologists who study happiness define it as a sense of overall well-being. It's not going around thinking nice thoughts or being a Pollyanna all the time; it's simple contentment. You enjoy your life. And you make the most of everything you can.

Loving marriages, family ties, and friendships predict happiness, as do spirituality and self-esteem. Hope is vital, too, as is the feeling that your life has meaning.

My first marriage lasted twenty-five years. As the marriage was falling apart, I wasn't getting a lot of warm fuzzies from the relationship, but that was okay. I made a conscious effort to put my energy into my career, my children, and doing the very best job I could as a mom and a medical examiner. That's what gave my life meaning and where I found my happiness.

Happiness may have a strong genetic component, according to many researchers. People seem to be born with a certain capacity for contentment, and no matter what happens in their lives, they eventually gravitate back to whatever degree of happiness comes naturally to them. Even so, researchers now believe happiness is something you can work at. It's a matter of figuring out what positive activities you can do and what positive emotions you can express every day.

How Not to Die from Negativity and Other Health-Eroding Emotions

Clearly, emotions play a profound part in bringing on disease and helping to combat it. That's why one of the most powerful secrets of how not to die is to guard your mental health. Be aware of a persistently gloomy mood, hopelessness, irritability, fears and anxieties that don't let up, or unrelenting stress, so you can get help when you need it. Learn how to manage pressure points in your life. Most of all, minimize negativity and cultivate happiness. This doesn't mean you have to be perpetually cheery to be happy or healthy; it means navigating life's rough spots with some positive strategies, and learning to feel content no matter the outcome. All of this is easier said than done, of course, but let me offer up some specific suggestions for how to do it.

Find Your Pony

Many people might think that being in a room full of dead people every day would be a downer. Sure, there's a real "gross" factor to my job—people die of infections, there are maggots, and things are slimy. A lot of people don't like dealing with corpses and lawyers on a daily basis, and the word "morgue" can conjure up a host of unpleasant emotions. And in my line of work, there are no hugs from happy patients. But I feel like I have one of the best jobs in the world because every day I'm reminded of how fragile life is, and it makes me live more fully. I also get to find the truth behind someone's death, and this helps the living in so many different ways.

Happy people are engaged in activities and careers that make them happy, and that menu is different for everyone. My parents weren't wealthy—my dad was a butcher and my mother was a homemaker—but they valued education. I was able to go to college and med school, where I found my niche in a career I enjoy, and so I have a great outlook on my job even though I work daily with death. I liken it to the familiar story of the two little boys who were both put into a room full of horse manure as an experiment by a psychiatrist. The first little boy simply plopped down and began to cry hopelessly and helplessly. The second little boy, as soon as he was placed in the room, began digging through the manure with both hands as fast as he could. This went on for quite awhile,

while the psychiatrist secretly watched. Finally, the psychiatrist interrupted the little boy to ask him what he was doing. The boy responded cheerfully, "With all this manure, I know there's got to be a pony in here somewhere!"

The way you look at the world will help your outlook. When your life looks more like a room full of manure than the mansion you've been dreaming about, don't just sit down and feel sorry for yourself. Get up and start digging. There's got to be a pony in there somewhere.

Cultivate Gratefulness

I see people every day who didn't know their last meal would be their last, that every action they'd taken or everything they tried was part of some finite number that would run out. I live with the reminder that we're all here temporarily, and so I'm grateful for life every day.

Being grateful is one of the keys to real happiness. The people whom I admire the most are those who are grateful for whatever they have, no matter what their lot in life. I've known people who've experienced terrible circumstances, from becoming paralyzed in an accident to losing a child, yet they can still manage a smile, a kind word, or an appreciation for life. These people are heroes to me.

Gratitude research suggests that feelings of thankfulness have tremendous positive value in helping us cope with daily problems, especially stress. Grateful people tend to be more optimistic, a characteristic that boosts the immune system and increases longevity. At the University of Pennsylvania, researchers asked volunteers to write down three good things that happened to them each day and why they thought they happened—and to do this every night for a week. This exercise, aimed at increasing gratitude, made people feel happier and less depressed—feelings that continued for months. It sure makes sense to pay attention to the good things in your life if you want to be happy.

So every now and then, consider the things or people you're grateful for.

Write them down if it suits you, keep a gratitude journal, or just talk to yourself in an appreciative way.

Shake the Blues with Professional Help

What's in your head has a direct effect on what's going on in your body. Depression or anxiety can hurt your health, and if you're being treated for an illness, your recovery will be better and faster if your mood is addressed. If you're unsure where to go for help, talk to your family doctor and see whether you can get help, either through medicines or counseling. Here are some additional resources:

- Mental health specialists, such as psychiatrists, psychologists, social workers, or mental health counselors
- Veterans hospitals and clinics (if you're eligible)
- Community mental health centers
- Hospital psychiatry departments and outpatient clinics
- Mental health programs at universities or medical schools
- State hospital outpatient clinics
- Family services, social agencies, or clergy
- Peer support groups
- Private clinics and facilities
- Employee assistance programs
- Local medical and/or psychiatric societies

Stress Less

Sometimes I get so busy and bogged down at work and with day-to-day living that it's hard to juggle everything. In addition to my morgue duties, I have the responsibilities of being chief medical examiner, filming the TV show, and taking care of my family. At the end of an autopsy day, I toss my protective clothing into a special trash can, throw my scrubs into a laundry basket, wash my hands, and get into my street clothes. I generally leave the morgue at 5:30 p.m. because I have to be home by seven most nights to get dinner ready and spend time with Mark and our sons. As much as possible, we try to eat dinner as a family and exchange stories about our days.

I never give up on a case, but I do what I can to strike a healthy balance between my job and my personal life. Having two doctors in the family makes life hectic, but we always manage to go to our sons' school events and football and basketball games. I cook dinner most nights, and my family's favorite is my lasagna, but I don't cook after a day of autopsies. Not because of the disturbing sights or smells, but because I've been standing and cutting all day, and cooking is more standing and cutting. We usually end up ordering takeout, or having a quick salad.

I think it's important to separate work and family life to reduce stress, and research bears this out. Several years ago, researchers at Michigan State University found that people who set boundaries between work and home were more connected to their families and have less conflict than those who integrate the two. Their research also suggested that people with these clear boundaries are happier.

Stress definitely has a negative impact on happiness. Whenever I feel stressed out, I take time for myself, which usually means going for a run. It clears my head and takes the edge off my day. An avalanche of studies shows that exercise is a great antidote for depression and anxiety.

Or I find someone to talk to. Turning to others helps me in times of stress. Accomplishing simple goals relaxes me, too, like getting all the laundry done in one weekend and not seeing it piled up in my laundry room on Monday morning.

Find a healthy outlet for stress. If it's not exercising, carve out some distraction-free quiet time to meditate or relax. Unplug the phone, order in dinner—whatever you need to do to find some quiet time. Or as I do, find a confidant. When you're stressed and focused too much in one direction, you need someone to vent to. Keeping things bottled up can wreck your immune system and wear you down.

I believe, too, that we're prepared to deal better with stress with the right attitude. It's not the stressful event that promotes illness, but our attitude toward that event. Two people faced with exactly the same stressor can react in almost opposite ways: One person may see a disaster, and the other may see an opportunity. Which would you rather be?

Reconnect with Nature

My older son, Alex, loves to work in the garden. He has planted a pumpkin garden every spring since he was eight years old. But now away at college, he wasn't able to finish his garden this year. The fact that it rained during his spring break hindered the project, too. Mark and I volunteered to finish it for him, and it was fun and invigorating.

Planting, digging, mulching, mowing, and other gardening activities can be therapeutic if you enjoy them. They're good for your heart, keep you mobile, and lengthen life. In a Seattle study, gardening for just an hour a week appeared to lower the risk of sudden cardiac death by 66 percent. I think a special relationship occurs when people nurture plants. Enjoying the outdoors, getting your fingers dirty, and seeing the rewards of something beautiful you've tended can help you live a healthier, less-crazed life.

A Smile a Day Keeps the M.E. Away

People tell me I have an engaging smile. I guess it's because I'm thinking happy thoughts most of the time, and the emotion I have on the inside easily comes out on the outside. Sometimes my smile is misinterpreted, and people think I'm smiling inappropriately. This can be a problem when you work in the morgue! When I was in fifth grade, my teacher would whack me on my back with a yardstick, saying, "Get that stupid look off your face!" All I was doing was smiling. It's just my natural look.

Most of us understand that emotions have corresponding physical counterparts. Fear, for example, can provoke a stress response in which the heart and breathing quicken. Such responses form a link between emotions and health. But how much control do we have over our emotional states? Are emotions simply automatic reactions, or can we force ourselves to be happy? Can we truly "put on a happy face"?

Psychologists say that our minds and bodies react to changes in our facial expressions. In experiments, smiling and looking happy not only made people feel happy but also caused their bodies to react as if they were happy. So smile! It might just put you in a better mood.

Laugh Yourself Healthy

I love to laugh, although not a lot of gallows humor goes on in the morgue. We try to show respect for the individuals we are autopsying. We may laugh and joke, but it's usually about one another and not about the dead. The other day, we poked a little fun at Steve Hansen, one of my investigators. He's always been jealous of the fact that as schoolkids, some were chosen to be crossing guards, and he wasn't. His childhood angst came to the surface when he found out that one of our morgue staff members had served as a crossing guard. Once this long-repressed, unfulfilled wish was discovered, one of our secretaries created a picture of a properly attired eleven-year-old crossing guard and pasted Steve's bearded sixty-year-old face on it. We had a good laugh over that prank. I don't think the dead would mind our jokes about one another and would probably laugh, too, if they could.

Laughing is therapeutic. It produces a relaxation response. Your blood pressure, heart rate, and muscle tension all drop below normal. It's a painkiller, too, because it stimulates the brain to produce more feel-good endorphins. One experiment in which people watched a humorous videotape showed that laughter spurs the production of antibodies in the upper respiratory tract that protect against infection. And another study found that laughing is a good workout: By laughing ten to fifteen minutes a day, you can burn up to forty calories.

What can you do to laugh more? Watch comedies, read the funnies, or hang out with people who make you laugh. Laugh often and much, including at yourself.

Turn Obstacles into Opportunities

I've had a blessed life, but it hasn't always been rosy. I've suffered setbacks like anyone else. My first marriage ended in divorce, my dad died a lingering, painful death from colon cancer, and I've been told twice that I probably had cancer. I also tried for eight years to get pregnant with my first child. (Had I not gotten pregnant, I knew I could adopt. I chose to think in terms of all my options.)

But I finally did get pregnant. During my pregnancy, I cruised right along with no major health problems until—boom—my face became paralyzed from a reactivation of chicken pox (shingles). I could barely close my eyes, I drooled at times, and, worst of all, I couldn't smile normally. Doctors gave me only a 30 percent chance that I'd regain use of my facial nerves. I hoped for the best and made peace with the prognosis.

Most people can't feel positive emotions at will. But you can approach events in a way that gets them going, then let momentum take over. I made a decision to see the positive when faced with bad news about my pregnancy. From everything the obstetrician had told me, I was expecting a healthy baby boy. But when the results of prenatal screening tests came back, I was informed that my son might be born with Down's syndrome. At that moment, I didn't fully comprehend what it meant. I just knew that if the Down's diagnosis was correct, my son was going to have challenges, and that this wasn't going to be the idyllic version of family life I had imagined. After contemplating this information for a few hours, I decided to relax, get my hair done, and accept the situation. I didn't say, "What a mess I'm in," and become immobilized by it. Instead, I put my disappointment behind me and focused on the positives. I knew my son would be a loving child, because most Down's children are. I started to plan my life accordingly. As it turned out, I eventually regained full use of my facial nerves, and my son was not born with Down's (there was a calculation error in one of the screening tests).

You can whine, you can moan, or you can pity yourself, but ultimately nobody's life is perfect. It helps me to make peace with the fact that life rarely turns out the way I expect. And that's true whether it comes to health problems, relationships with people you care about, or even your hopes and dreams for your kids.

Embracing all of your life experiences—even the really painful ones—with the knowledge that something good inevitably will come out of them is what engenders happiness, contentment, and peace. If you keep a positive, rational attitude of "It's worth a try!" or "I accept the challenge!" and plow forward with a positive course of action, I believe good things will happen to you.

Explore More

My husband loves to go fishing, and I get seasick. A few summers ago, he planned a fishing trip for us to the Olympic Peninsula of Washington State, where he vacationed as a child. Mark's plan was to rent a boat and head out to the ocean to fish for salmon. The thought of this trip sent shivers down my spine. But my boys were so excited that there was no way I was going to let them know I'd rather test bulletproof vests than get in a small boat on choppy seas, early on a cold morning. I knew the trip meant a lot to them, and I wanted to share the experience. I made myself have a good attitude about the trip. I took medicine so I wouldn't get seasick. I read up on how to fish for salmon. And you know what? I had a wonderful time, and I can't wait to do it again.

I really believe that one of the paths to happiness is through pushing yourself out of your comfort zone. If you've always gone on the same vacation or read the same books, you'll never know if you're truly growing as a person. Researchers tell us that when we expose ourselves to new challenges, we build our knowledge and experience, which increases confidence, happiness, and well-being.

It takes a certain amount of effort, but have some new adventures a few times a year. I don't mean you have to swim the English Channel. Try a new hobby, eat something unfamiliar, or learn a new instrument. As I did with my fishing trip, shake off negative preconceptions, and be open to new experiences.

Get Restorative Rest

About every three days, I autopsy a suicide victim. There are many reasons why these tragic acts occur. In many suicides I see, there's a history of depression; in others, the suicide comes from out of the blue, an impulsive act with very little preceding depression. In many cases of impulsive suicide, there is a history of sleep deprivation.

One case I autopsied a few months ago was of Bret Nelson, an eighteen-year-old student who was good-looking with an athletic build. I particularly remember his long eyelashes. He was not having problems with school or friends. His family said he had always been awkward around women, but he had recently started dating a girl he really liked. After a few dates, though, she informed him that she no longer wanted to go out with him. He seemed to take it hard but not in a way that was disturbing. Then he started having trouble sleeping and went forty-eight to seventy-two hours straight without sleep. Sitting at the dinner table with his parents, Bret informed them that he was going to go out to the yard to kill himself. That he immediately did, with a gunshot wound to the head. The parents had a hard time accepting this as a suicide. They told me just three days earlier he was a normal boy with plans and dreams. Lack of sleep seems to be similar to alcohol, in that both dramatically decrease inhibitions that would normally keep us from self-destructive or violent acts.

Sleep disorders are common in those who suffer from depression. The vicious loop of worsening depression and more severe sleep loss can lead to disaster. One case I recall involved a man named Marcus Bennett, a forty-seven-year-old engineer who was found dead in his home. He had a bullet hole in his head, and there was a 9 mm revolver lying beside his body. Detectives verified that the gun belonged to Marcus and that he had talked about suicide in the past. These clues, plus the trajectory of the bullet, led me to rule that he had indeed died by his own hand.

Found at the scene, too, was an unused sleep apnea machine, used to supply gentle air pressure that keeps airways open while someone is sleeping. Sleep apnea, which I discussed in chapter 5 as a complication of obesity, is a serious condition that causes people to stop breathing repeatedly—in some cases, hundreds of times—during their sleep. It's linked not only to medical problems such as obesity, high blood pressure, and increased risk of heart failure, heart attack, and stroke, but also with mood disorders. Some research suggests that sleep apnea is associated with personality changes, irritability, mood swings, depression, and a poor quality of life.

Whether Marcus Bennett's sleep problems were the major factor in his depression or suicide, I'll never know. What I do know is that sleep deprivation can rob you of physical and mental well-being. In fact, when you habitually get less sleep than you need each night, your risk of having an accident or developing heart disease, cancer, diabetes, memory problems, or depression begins to increase.

There's a great deal of debate on how many hours of sleep we need a night, but as a general rule, if you tend to sleep late on weekends or always need an alarm to wake you, you might be sleep-deprived. To get a good night's sleep: Try going to bed at set time each night and get up at the same time each morning. Stay away from caffeine, nicotine, and alcohol, all of which can keep you awake. Alcohol robs the body of deep sleep. Have some relaxation rituals such as reading before you go to bed. Keep your bedroom a comfortable temperature. If you can't get to sleep, don't just lie there. Do something else, like reading or listening to music, until you feel drowsy. Music can relax the body, sometimes lulling you into sleep. If your sleeping problem continues, don't be embarrassed to see your doctor.

TURN THE TABLES: If You or Someone You Know Is Contemplating Suicide

If you're thinking about harming yourself, or know a person who is, tell someone who can help immediately.

- Call your doctor.
- Call 911 or go to a hospital emergency room to get immediate help, or ask a friend or family member to help you do these things.
- Call the toll-free, twenty-four-hour hotline of the National Suicide Prevention Lifeline at (800) 273-TALK (8255), TTY: (800) 799-4TTY (4889), to talk to a trained counselor.
- Make sure you or the suicidal person is not left alone.

Do Good to Feel Good

If I could write a prescription to encourage a lifetime of health and happiness, it might be this: "Help other people." In fact, one study in the *Journal of Health and Social Behavior* found that volunteer work can boost happiness, life satisfaction, self-esteem, sense of control over life, physical health, and mood.

Doing nice things for people without expectation of compensation gives me a lot of pleasure. It connects me to others, gives me a purpose, and makes me realize that I'm not so important. It's not that you have to go on a save-the-world crusade, either. I'm not out there curing cancer or creating world peace. I just try to give my all to my little circle of influence and the people in it. I show love for the people in my life. I treat people with respect and help them discover their self-worth. I try to develop greater empathy for those whose needs are different from my own. I do the very best I can every day at my job. I like to think that there's a ripple effect of these contributions, and that it will widen forever.

Everybody has something to give to this world, whether it's helping out at a spaghetti dinner, pledging money to a school booster club, or just performing your job well. Doing things for other people doesn't necessarily involve donating a lot of time, either. Much of it has to do with the way you treat people, like saying a kind word to the bank teller or being a phenomenal spouse and parent. When what you do in your daily life for others speaks to your heart, you'll feel happier.

Share Your Story

I love telling the story of how my husband and I reunited and recently married. I met Mark thirty years ago while we were both in medical school. We were in love, and he asked me to marry him. I said no. He was Protestant, I was Catholic. He wanted to live on the West Coast, I wanted to stay in the Midwest. I was young and stupid and thought those things mattered. We both went our separate ways and married others, though we stayed in periodic contact professionally. My marriage ended in divorce, and Mark's wife passed away from ovarian cancer. When we saw each other again after many years, our eyes locked and sparks flew. In that moment, we knew we were meant to be together. Mark surprised me with a marriage proposal in a seaplane flying over the Puget Sound, and in 2006, we were married on Amelia Island. Our romance had come full circle. Whenever I think of that story, or tell it, I always get positive, warm, and loving feelings.

A study published in the *Journal of Personality and Social Psychology* found that telling others about positive experiences increases the positive emotion connected with the event. And each time the good news is shared, positive emotions build even more. There's a wonderful lesson here: Recall and talk about positive things in your life. Don't be afraid to share good news. All of this brings about happiness.

Heal Loneliness

Some of my cases are like a locked room. No matter how much I pound on the door, I'll never be able to see inside or know the true chain of events that brings someone to my morgue. But in the case of Phillip Greenlaw, age forty-three, I suspect that loneliness, as much as anything else, is what killed him.

Phillip's lifeless body was found by a maintenance man on the bedroom floor of his small condominium in St. Cloud. Twenty-eight blue pills were lying on the dresser. His landlord said Phillip was an unemployed hotel concierge who lived by himself. He had recently been fired from a local Italian restaurant, and his wife and three children had long ago left him. Phillip had been depressed about his marriage and the recent downturn in his job situation. On top of everything else, he had been drinking too much.

Signs of his depression and drinking were evident in the autopsy. I saw a well-healed horizontal scar on his left wrist, indicating a previous suicide attempt. He also suffered from "dilated cardiomyopathy," a common form of heart muscle disease. In dilated cardiomyopathy, the heart chambers are abnormally distended. Up to 30 percent of cases of dilated cardiomyopathy are linked to heavy drinking. After years of alcohol abuse, the heart can be weakened by alcohol's toxic effect on its muscle cells.

The blue pills were identified as diphenhydramine, the active ingredient in several over-the-counter antihistamines and sleep aids. Toxicology tests on Phillip's body revealed a lethal level of diphenhydramine. I estimated that he couldn't have lived longer than several hours after taking them. Exactly why Phillip took the pills was uncertain, and I ruled the manner of death as suicide.

This case reminded me that loneliness can exact a heavy toll. Most people experience feelings of loneliness from time to time, but for people like Phillip

Greenlaw, it can become a chronic problem that can seriously affect physical and mental health. Loneliness is a major precipitant of depression and alcoholism, and increases the risk of suicide.

If you feel lonely all the time and need someone with whom you can share your innermost thoughts, please do something about it. Feeling lonely doesn't mean that you're a failure or that there's something wrong with you, but it's a sign you may have important needs that are not being met. We're social animals, and we all need the companionship of others to function at our best. Social contact staves off depression and stress and boosts the immune system. Plenty of research shows that people with family, friends, partners, or pets live longer than those who don't.

My mother lives alone. She's eighty-eight and I'd love to inherit her longevity. Part of her secret is that she talks to her best friend by phone every single day, and her kids call her every day. Reach out to people you know. I bet friends and relatives who haven't heard from you in a long time will be happy to reestablish contact, and the interaction will make you feel better. Look for ways to get involved with people as you go about your daily life. Join a club or sign up for a class. Taking part in activities that interest you will make it more likely you'll meet people with whom you have something in common. If you have difficulty dealing with your feelings of loneliness on your own, perhaps a counselor can help you work through them.

Marry Happy

The closest relationship most adults ever develop is marriage. Marriage may be one of the best things you can do—but only if it's a good one. Researchers say that happily married men and women report higher levels of life satisfaction than do subjects who are divorced or who never married. Marriage affects immunity and physical health, too. When we're under stress, angered, or depressed by divorce, separation, or widowhood, the number of immune cells that protect us against disease is reduced. A troubled union hurts health, too. In one study, scientists at the Ohio State University observed that blister wounds healed more slowly following marital conflicts than wounds in couples who were more loving and supportive toward each other. The quality of a relationship matters in terms of good health.

What makes a quality marriage?

To me, a quality marriage is like an ice cream sundae. I'm the scoop of vanilla ice cream, my kids are the chocolate sauce, and my husband is the whipped cream with the cherry on top. If you're more like pickled cabbage, you can layer on all the fixings, but you're not going to have a good dessert. You're going to sour the taste of everything. So a quality marriage starts with you, being happy with yourself, as that scoop of ice cream from which all good things build.

Granted, I'm no marriage counselor, but my years in the morgue have given me a unique perspective on the human condition. I know that the most significant connection we can have is with our partners. They can be our lovers, best friends, confidants, social partners, and financial partners. When you have a loving, supportive partner, you feel secure in knowing there's someone on your side, someone who—when push comes to shove—is there for you. The things partners do to connect and show their commitment—touching, hugging, listening, supporting—all trigger the release of endorphins that give you a sense of peace and tranquillity. If you have not yet found or have lost your soul mate, research shows that these endorphins are also released with close relationships with other human beings, and even with our pets. When you get—and stay—connected, your life becomes less stressful.

In the end, it's clear that the factors affecting our life spans are far more subtle and complex than had previously been thought. If you wish to live a long life, it isn't only a matter of eating the right foods, exercising, not smoking, or driving with care. You've also got to have the right attitude. So look on the bright side. It's another powerful strategy for how not to die.

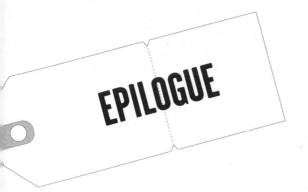

EPILOGUE

Lessons on How Not to Die

After I finished the last chapter of this book, it was my weekend to cover the morgue. It was a slow weekend for homicides, but a bad weekend for preventable deaths. Take, for instance, William Craig. He could be a poster boy for this book. He was thirty-six years old, weighed 389 pounds, smoked, and was told he had high blood pressure eight years ago but had decided to stop taking his hypertensive medications seven and a half years ago because he "felt fine."

William was so heavy he had a hard time breathing. He had also been diagnosed with sleep apnea. He was brought to the morgue on a reinforced gurney (recently added to our standard equipment because of the increase in the morbidly obese coming through the morgue) and placed on a reinforced special autopsy table.

While I was reading his history and deciding if I really needed to do an autopsy, I discovered another behavior that's a sure road to my morgue: He abused his prescription pain medications. What started out as treatment for sore knees and wear-and-tear arthritis from being so overweight became a full-fledged addiction to pain meds.

Ultimately, the toxicology revealed he died from an accidental overdose of his pain medication, but I also determined at autopsy that he would not have been long for this world anyway. His heart was enlarged and the heart muscle wall thickened from the effects of hypertension and obesity. He also had narrowing of his coronary arteries by atherosclerotic plaque, as well as early emphysema due to cigarette smoking. When talking to his family, I found out that William had a long history of unhappiness over a failed relationship ten years earlier. Was that unhappiness the root of all his bad lifestyle choices? I'll never know. If he had read and heeded some of the advice in this book, there's little doubt he wouldn't have been there on that particular Saturday, spending the day in the morgue with me.

My new mantra in the morgue is, "Here's another one who should have read my book." It's my way of noting that yet another death could have been avoided. The advice I give in this book is simple, but it can have a profound effect on your longevity. How not to die really boils down to a set of basic instructions.

Lesson #1: Know your numbers.

You'll live a longer and healthier life when your body mass index (BMI) is under 25. It may be possible to have a full life span with a somewhat higher BMI (25–29) if you stay in good shape, but in no event should you tolerate a BMI over 29. Aiming for 24 should be your goal. The adverse health effects of obesity are multiple and avoidable.

Know your blood glucose (blood sugar level). The consequences of elevated blood glucose are not only eventual plaque formation and narrowing of the blood vessels, particularly the coronary arteries, but also damage to your nerves, kidneys, eyes, and immune system. Millions of people are walking around with diabetes, with its effects already ravaging their bodies. Diabetes is sometimes not detected until something terrible happens, like a heart attack, stroke, or kidney failure. Seize the initiative and have this simple test!

Check your blood pressure early and check it often. Just about every drugstore I walk into has an automated blood pressure monitor, so use it. If your blood pressure is greater than 130/85, bring the information to a physician and take action. High blood pressure is a silent killer. You can feel great right up until the moment you die; I see this virtually every day. Hypertension is one of the leading cause of kidney failure (being on dialysis is no fun), and causes enlargement of the heart, accelerated atherosclerosis in your arteries, and sudden hemorrhages in the brain (hemorrhagic stroke), all of which can have sudden death as their first symptom.

The last numbers that are essential to know are your lipid profile: total cholesterol, LDL cholesterol (the bad one, which should be low), and HDL cholesterol (the good one, which should be high). Heart disease, particularly due to atherosclerotic plaque buildup (narrowed coronary arteries), and ischemic strokes are major causes of premature death. Cholesterol-lowering drugs are a major success story in modern medicine. They're inexpensive, well tolerated, and extremely effective. Take advantage of this great medical advance.

Lesson #2: Listen to your body.

If something doesn't feel right or you have an unusual pain that causes concern, pay attention to it. See your doctor and find an answer. Be proactive about your health and seek help early. Get regular physicals and have appropriate screening tests.

Lesson #3: Use as directed.

So many things in life come with instructions—and for good reason. Instructions tell us how to do things right so we won't get hurt or injure others. To increase your odds of living a long and fulfilling life: Take your medicine as directed, follow your doctor's orders, and obey posted and written rules.

Lesson #4: Practice good hygiene.

This advice isn't just your mother nagging you, either. Studies show that the more often you wash your hands, the less likely you are to get sick. Keeping your hands clean is one of the best ways to avoid illness. Along those same lines, use condoms when needed, since HIV is largely transmitted through sexual contact. Nearly 60 percent of AIDS cases diagnosed since 1981 could have been prevented by using condoms.

Lesson #5: Drive carefully.

The tendency to take chances on the highway that can land you in traffic court can just as easily land you in the morgue. Wear a seat belt when driving and a helmet when bike riding. Don't drink or do drugs and drive. Observe all rules of the road.

Lesson #6: Just say no.

Smoking is one of the best ways to ensure you'll wind up in the morgue. Get help to quit, if necessary. A little bit of alcohol may be healthy, but more than moderate amounts are not. Don't mess with recreational and illicit drugs, and don't abuse prescription drugs. The less you put of these things in your body, the greater your chances of being around for a long time to come.

Lesson #7: Watch your step.

Think about the consequences of your actions. Sure, I see some unavoidable accidents in the morgue, but a large percentage could have been prevented, and that includes most car accidents. I have the choice of only five manners of death on the death certificate: homicide, suicide, natural, accident, and undetermined. If I could add another, it would be "stupidity." It's difficult to say a cause of death is an accident when the decedent's death was clearly avoidable if he or she had applied a little thinking to the situation.

Lesson #8: Have a good time.

What's important isn't whether you got all of the food stains off your blouse or shirt. It's whether you had a good time at the picnic, the candlelit dinner, or the ice cream store with your kids. If you enjoyed yourself, then the experience was well worth it, whether your clothes looked good afterward or not. As you go through life, have fun and get a daily dose of vitamin H. Humor—through laughter and smiling—eases the burdens of life.

Lesson #9: Don't go it alone.

Relationships are important to me. Life revolves around them, and it shows in our health. People who maintain close relationships live longer and more healthily. Tap into the healing network of family and friends, neighbors and colleagues, so that when stressful, difficult times come, you'll have supportive people all around. It may sound corny, but caring for others helps us care for ourselves and brings added meaning to our lives.

Lesson #10: Remember what matters.

There's one thing that I'd like my kids to remember about me: I cared. I cared about my family, and I always put them first. We all need to clarify what's truly important and set priorities that make sense for us. When all is said and done, it's not how many years you live, it's what you do with those years.

Life has its challenges at times, and death is inevitable. We just don't have to help it along.

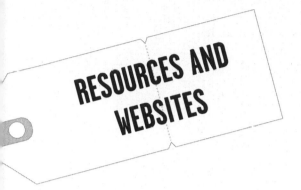
RESOURCES AND WEBSITES

General Health Information

Agency for Healthcare Research and Quality
U.S. Department of Health and
    Human Services
(800) 358-9295
www.ahrq.gov

American Academy of Family Physicians
www.familydoctor.org

American Medical Association
(800) 621-8335
www.ama-assn.org

Centers for Disease Control and Prevention
U.S. Department of Health and
    Human Services
www.cdc.gov
www.healthfinder.gov

(Healthfinder can direct you to medical journals and other publications, clearinghouses, databases, hotlines, medical research, support groups, organizations, and libraries.)

MedicineNet.com
www.medicinenet.com

National Women's Health Information Center
U.S. Department of Health and
    Human Services
(800) 994-9662
www.4women.gov

Alcohol and Drug Abuse

National Clearinghouse for Alcohol and Drug Information
Substance Abuse and Mental Health
    Services Administration
U.S. Department of Health and
    Human Services
(800) 729-6686
www.health.org

National Institute on Alcohol Abuse and Alcoholism
National Institutes of Health
U.S. Department of Health and
    Human Services
(301) 443-3860
www.niaaa.nih.gov

National Institute on Drug Abuse
National Institutes of Health
U.S. Department of Health and
    Human Services
(301) 443-1124
www.drugabuse.gov

Cancer

American Cancer Society
(800) ACS-2345
www.cancer.org

Cancer Information Service
National Cancer Institute
National Institutes of Health
U.S. Department of Health and
    Human Services
(800) 422-6237
www.cancer.gov

Depression

American Psychological Association
(800) 374-2721 or (202) 336-5500
www.apa.org

National Institute of Mental Health
National Institutes of Health
U.S. Department of Health and
    Human Services
(301) 443-4513
www.nimh.nih.gov

Diabetes

American Diabetes Association
ATTN: National Call Center
(800) DIABETES or (800) 342-2383
www.diabetes.org

**Lower Extremity Amputation
Prevention Program (LEAP)**
Bureau of Primary Health Care
Health Resources and Services
    Administration
U.S. Department of Health and
    Human Services
(888) 275-4772
www.hrsa.gov/leap

**National Institute of Diabetes and
Digestive and Kidney Diseases**
National Institutes of Health
U.S. Department of Health and
    Human Services
(301) 496-3583
www.niddk.nih.gov

Forensic Pathology

**National Association of Medical
Examiners**
www.thename.org

Heart Disease

American Heart Association
(800) AHA-USA-1 or (800) 242-8721
www.americanheart.org

Hospitals

The Joint Commission
(630) 792-5000
www.jointcommission.org

Obesity and Nutrition

American Dietetic Association
(800) 877-1600
www.eatright.org

Weight Control Information Network
National Institutes of Health
U.S. Department of Health and
    Human Services
(877) 946-4627
www.win.niddk.nih.gov

Smoking

American Lung Association
(212) 315-8700 or (800) LUNGUSA (to
    contact the American Lung
    Association nearest you)
www.lungusa.org

Cancer Information Service
National Cancer Institute
National Institutes of Health
U.S. Department of Health and
    Human Services
(800) 422-6237
www.cancer.gov

Stroke

**National Institute of Neurological
Disorders and Stroke**
National Institutes of Health
U.S. Department of Health and
    Human Services
(800) 352-9424
www.ninds.nih.gov

National Stroke Association
9707 East Easter Lane
Centennial, CO 80112
(800) STROKES or (800) 787-6537
www.stroke.org

Travel and Tropical Medicine

**American Society of Tropical
Medicine and Hygiene**
(847) 480-9592
www.astmh.org

**Centers for Disease Control
and Prevention**
U.S. Department of Health and
    Human Services
www.cdc.gov

**International Association for Medical
Assistance to Travelers**
(716) 754-4883
www.iamat.org

SELECTED BIBLIOGRAPHY

1. Doctor Dread

Agency for Healthcare Research and Quality (AHRQ). 2003. *Men: Stay healthy at any age—your checklist for health* (booklet).
———. 2003. *Pocket guide to good health for adults* (booklet).
———. 2007. *The guide to clinical preventive services.*
Prochazka, A. V., et al. 2005. "Support of evidence-based guidelines for the annual physical examination: A survey of primary care providers." *Archives of Internal Medicine* 165: 1347–52.

2. Deadly Prescriptions

Agency for Healthcare Research and Quality (AHRQ). 2000. *20 tips to prevent medical errors* (booklet).
Bates, D. W., et al. 1998. "Effect of computerized physician order entry and a team intervention on prevention of serious medication errors." *Journal of the American Medical Association* 280: 1311–16.

Bolland, M. J., et al. 2008. "Vascular events in healthy older women receiving calcium supplements: Randomized controlled trial." *British Medical Journal* 336: 262–66.

Brunner, E. 2006. "Oily fish and omega 3 fat supplements." *British Medical Journal* 332: 739–40.

Burr, M. L. 2007. "Secondary prevention of CHD in UK men: The diet and reinfarction trial and its sequel." *The Proceedings of the Nutrition Society* 66: 9–15.

Gardinier, P., et al. 2007. "Factors associated with herbal therapy use by adults in the United States." *Alternative Therapies in Health and Medicine* 13: 22–29.

Velicer, C. M., and C. M. Ulrich. 2008. "Vitamin and mineral supplement use among U.S. adults after cancer diagnosis: A systematic review." *Journal of Clinical Oncology* 26: 665–73.

3. Code Blue

Hayward, R. A., and T. P. Hofer. 2001. "Estimating hospital deaths due to medical errors." *Journal of the American Medical Association* 286: 415–20.

4. Highway to the Morgue

Garavaglia, J., et al. 2003. "Seven hundred fifty-three consecutive deaths in a level I trauma center: The argument for injury prevention." *The Journal of Trauma* 54: 66–70.

5. Dead Weight

Rucker, D., et al. 2007. "Long term pharmacotherapy for obesity and overweight: Updated meta-analysis." *The British Medical Journal* 335: 1194–99.

Sears, D. 2006. Fatty liver. www.eMedicine.com.

Uwaifo, G. I. 2006. Obesity. www.eMedicine.com.

Wood, S. 2008. "Increased fitness associated with 50% to 70% reductions in all-cause mortality." www.medscape.com/medscapetoday.

6. Last Call

Dynamed. 2007. "Alcohol intoxication." www.DynamicMedical.com.

———. 2008. "Alcohol use disorder." www.DynamicMedical.com.

7. Dying to Get High

Dynamed. 2008. "Opiate dependence." www.DynamicMedical.com.
———. 2008. "Cocaine abuse." www.DynamicMedical.com.

8. Up in Smoke: Risking Life and Lung

Aldington, S., et al. 2007. "Effects of cannabis on pulmonary structure, function and symptoms." *Thorax* 62: 1058–63.
Benowitz, Neal L. 2003. "Tobacco." In *Cecil Textbook of Medicine,* 22 ed., ed. L. Goldman and D. Ausiello.
Marcus, B. H., et al. 1999. "The efficacy of exercise as an aid for smoking cessation in women: A randomized controlled trial." *Archives of Internal Medicine* 159: 1229–34.
Mariolis, P., et al. 2006. "Tobacco use among adults—United States." *Morbidity and Mortality Weekly Report* 55: 1145–48.
Mehra, R., et al. 2006. "The association between marijuana smoking and lung cancer: A systematic review." *Archives of Internal Medicine* 166: 1359–67.

9. Everyday Dangers

American Medical Association. 1997. Household safety. www.ama-assn.org.
National Safety Council. Odds of dying. www.nsc.org/research/odds.aspx.

10. Man, Oh Man!

Testorff, K. 2005. "Another dumb trick." *Sea and Shore* www.safetycenter.navy.mil/media/seashore/issues/spring05/anotherdumb.htm.

11. Permanent Vacation

Kop, W. J., et al. 2003. "Risk factors for myocardial infarction during vacation travel." *Psychosomatic Medicine* 65: 396–401.

12. Longevity Rx

Brummett, B. H., et al. 2006. "Prediction of all-cause mortality by the Minnesota Multiphasic Personality Inventory Optimism-Pessimism Scale scores: Study of a college sample during a 40-year follow-up period." *Mayo Clinic Proceedings* 81: 1541–44.

Buchowski, M. S., et al. 2007. "Energy expenditure of genuine laughter." *International Journal of Obesity (London)* 31: 131–37.

Das, S., and J. H. O'Keefe. 2006. "Behavioral cardiology: Recognizing and addressing the profound impact of psychosocial stress on cardiovascular health." *Current Atherosclerosis Reports* 8: 111–18.

Dillon, K. M., et al. 1985–86. "Positive emotional states and enhancement of the immune system." *International Journal of Psychiatry in Medicine* 15: 13–18.

Editor. 2005. "Sleep: Understanding the basics." EMedicineHealth.com.

Gable, S. L., et al. 2004. "What do you do when things go right? The intrapersonal and interpersonal benefits of sharing positive events." *Journal of Personality and Social Psychology* 87: 228–45.

Hassed, C. 2001. "How humour keeps you well." *Australian Family Physician* 30: 25–28.

Hawkley, L. C., and J. T. Cacioppo. 2003. "Loneliness and pathways to disease." *Brain Behavior and Immunity* 17 Suppl. no. 1: S98–S105.

Hershberger, P. J. 2005. "Prescribing happiness: Positive psychology and family medicine." *Family Medicine* 37: 630–34.

Jennings, L. B. 1997. "Potential benefits of pet ownership in health promotion." *Journal of Holistic Nursing* 15: 358–72.

Kiecolt-Glaser, J. K., et al. 2005. "Hostile marital interactions, proinflammatory cytokine production, and wound healing." *Archives of General Psychiatry* 62: 1377–84.

Lemaitre, R. N., et al. 1999. "Leisure-time physical activity and the risk of primary cardiac arrest." *Archives of Internal Medicine* 159: 686–90.

Thoits, P. A., and L. N. Hewitt. 2001. "Volunteer work and well-being." *Journal of Health and Social Behavior* 42: 115–31.

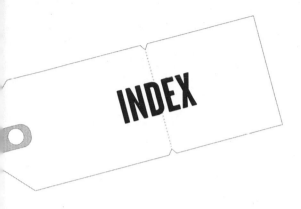

INDEX

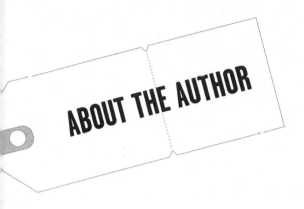

ABOUT THE AUTHOR

Jan C. Garavaglia, M.D. (a.k.a. Dr. G), is the chief medical examiner for the District Nine Medical Examiner Office covering Orange and Osceola counties in Florida and has been a forensic pathologist for twenty years.

A graduate of the St. Louis University School of Medicine, Dr. Garavaglia completed her internship in internal medicine and residency in pathology at the University Hospitals in St. Louis, Missouri. She then completed a fellowship in forensic pathology at the Dade County Medical Examiner Office in Miami, Florida. She is certified by the American Board of Pathology in anatomic, clinical, and forensic pathology.

Prior to joining the office in Florida, Dr. Garavaglia was a medical examiner at the Bexar County Forensic Science Center in San Antonio, Texas, for ten years. While there she also served as a clinical assistant professor for the department of pathology at the University of Texas Health Science Center at San Antonio and as a member of their Graduate Faculty Council for the Graduate School of Biomedical Science. She has also worked as a medical examiner in Jacksonville, Florida, and the metropolitan Atlanta area.

Dr. Garavaglia is a member of the National Association of Medical Examiners and the American Academy of Forensic Sciences, and is on the editorial board of the *American Journal of Forensic Medicine and Pathology*. She is a recipient of community service awards for her work in forensic pathology in San Antonio, Texas, and Orange County, Florida.

In addition, Dr. Garavaglia has given innumerable presentations and lectures at various institutions and has been published in scientific media such as the *Journal of Forensic Sciences, Journal of Trauma,* and *The American Journal of Forensic Medicine and Pathology*. She is the subject and host of the popular TV show *Dr. G.: Medical Examiner* on the Discovery Health channel and has appeared on *Larry King Live* and *The Oprah Winfrey Show*.

Dr. Garavaglia is married to Mark Wallace, M.D. They have three sons, Alex, Eric, and Luke.